CARING FOR THE LOW GERMAN MENNONITES

JUDITH C. KULIG

Caring for the Low German Mennonites

How Religious Beliefs and Practices Influence Health Care

PURICH BOOKS

Purich Books, an imprint of UBC Press
2029 West Mall, Vancouver, BC V6T 1Z2
www.purichbooks.ca

27 26 25 24 23 22 21 20 19 18 5 4 3 2 1

Printed in Canada on FSC-certified ancient-forest-free paper (100% post-consumer recycled) that is processed chlorine- and acid-free.

Library and Archives Canada Cataloguing in Publication

Kulig, Judith Celene, author
Caring for the Low German Mennonites : how religious beliefs and practices influence health care / Judith C. Kulig.

Includes bibliographical references and index.
Issued in print and electronic formats.
ISBN 978-0-7748-8015-2 (hardcover). – ISBN 978-0-7748-8017-6 (PDF).
ISBN 978-0-7748-8018-3 (EPUB). – ISBN 978-0-7748-8019-0 (Kindle)

1. Mennonites – Medical care – Canada. 2. Spiritual care (Medical care) – Canada. 3. Medical care – Canada. I. Title.

BX8118.5.K85 2018 362.1088'289771 C2018-901059-2
C2018-901060-6

Canadä

UBC Press gratefully acknowledges the financial support for our publishing program of the Government of Canada (through the Canada Book Fund), the Canada Council for the Arts, and the British Columbia Arts Council.

Printed and bound in Canada by Friesens
Set in Calibri and Sabon by Artegraphica Design Co. Ltd.
Copy editor: Deborah Kerr
Indexer: Stephen Ullstrom

To all the cheerleaders in my life
who have been with me along this journey.
Thanks for making sure I took a break, laughed,
and stopped to admire the beauty around me.

CONTENTS

Foreword / ix
John Janzen

Preface / xi

Acknowledgments / xv

Introduction / 3

1 A Brief History of the Low German Mennonites / 21

2 Health and Illness / 39

3 Women's Health / 55

4 Death and Dying / 79

5 Mental Health / 93

Conclusion /109

Notes / 117

References / 121

Index / 129

FOREWORD

Scattered across the globe, some 350,000 Low German Mennonites speak their own language, called Plautdietsch, and adhere to a unique faith-based lifestyle. All are Anabaptists and many are descended from the Old Colony Mennonites who emigrated from Russia during the late nineteenth century to settle in Canada. In the 1920s, many moved on, leaving Canada to establish new homes, predominantly in Mexico.

This group is the subject of Judith Kulig's research. A well-known researcher of rural health issues, she has devoted some twenty years of her academic career to studying Low German (LG) Mennonites, with the intent of providing valuable information to both the Low German community and those who interact with it in a variety of professional and personal capacities. Her various studies, which are documented in this book, entailed visiting and interviewing hundreds of LG Mennonites. Her research focuses on their religious beliefs and practices as they relate to health and illness. Since 1995, Judith has travelled extensively and made many presentations to caregivers, health practitioners, and interest groups. Her research has met the challenge of gaining access to a distinct group that has traditionally preferred to isolate itself from the rest of society.

Judith has been persistent in the pursuit of better health care for LG Mennonites – care based on the findings of her field research. Her work demonstrates LG Mennonites' resiliency in addressing health issues after they gain access to and understanding of the available health options. With its abundance of well-documented research, this book provides a deeper understanding of the Low German Mennonite community. Practitioners who care for members of this group will find it an invaluable resource.

John Janzen, retired Low German coordinator for Mennonite Central Committee Canada

PREFACE

LingLing and I walk through the field to take in the view of the Bustillos Valley spread before us. The day has just begun, and the peacefulness of dawn has not yet been broken. The mountains are blue in the morning light, tinted with the pink glow of sunrise. To our left, an Old Colony Mennonite woman, dressed in black, her head covered with a traditional scarf, walks in the fields. The red earth has been planted for the year. We can hear roosters crowing and the sound of agricultural equipment as the farmers begin their work for the day. To our right lie more fields, the irrigation system clearly visible at the ends of the rows to flood the crops.

I vividly remember walking every morning with LingLing (HaiYan) Fan, at that time a graduate student I was supervising, to take in the sky with its beautiful pink dawns and the view of the mountains beyond the seemingly endless rows of planted fields. In the mornings when we stood there, it was so utterly peaceful.

To a casual observer, the Bustillos Valley is simply another agricultural area in Mexico, but it also represents one stage in the historically and socially significant migration of a unique religious group – the

Low German Mennonites. Settling there and carving out a new life must have been difficult. The women's long, dark dresses would have been hot and heavy. There would have been many new things to learn: the agricultural properties of the soil, how to determine which crops would flourish, and how to manage the unfamiliar currency. Despite all the challenges, the Low German Mennonites succeeded as farmers and entrepreneurs, eventually founding the Mennonite Museum, which is now a tourist destination in Ciudad Cuauhtémoc. As a community, they volunteered to help Mexicans in times of drought and disaster. Importantly, their links to Canada persisted through relatives and friends, despite the physical distance and philosophical differences. For example, during a trip to Mexico, I met a sister of one of my Canadian research assistants, as well as relatives of individuals whom we had interviewed in Canada. The world may be physically large, but when it comes to connections between people, it is really very small.

In 1995, when I supervised fourth-year nursing students as they completed a cultural assessment of Low German (LG) Mennonites in southern Alberta, I never imagined that studying this small religious community would dominate so much of my academic career and become a significant part of my rural health research program. After that initial contact, I undertook fieldwork in Belize, in Cuauhtémoc, Mexico, and in Durango Colony, Mexico, during which I conducted 15 interviews. In total, I have led four research studies: two solely in Alberta, one in Alberta and Manitoba, and the final one in Alberta, Manitoba, and Ontario. For these studies, we interviewed 217 LG Mennonites and 82 health and social service providers and others who care for this population, such as funeral directors and teacher aides. We tailored our research questions and approach to be respectful of LG Mennonite beliefs and principles. As in any project, we encountered challenges along the way, such as the concerns of ministers about interviewing their congregation, and I sometimes had difficulty in convincing LG Mennonites and historians that I was sincerely interested in learning about this group. There were also many rewards, such as the satisfaction of hearing respondents say that they now understood why their church or family held certain beliefs or that our questions had stimulated them to think about our questions even after the interview ended. Presenting our results to health providers, who had "ah-ha" moments when they recalled LG Mennonites whom they had cared for but not fully understood, was gratifying as well.

As a practising nurse, I had worked extensively with a variety of cultural groups, including several First Nations and Cambodian and Central American refugees. I had learned about their cultural backgrounds and developed bilingual health promotion materials to address their health issues. With this background in cross-cultural nursing, I already knew that diversity was an important part of our society. When I conducted my LG Mennonite studies, it became obvious, and was continually reinforced, that *religious* diversity is a key form of overall diversity and that it deserves attention in its own right. We typically associate religious diversity with immigrants or refugees, rather than with groups that have a long history in Canada, such as the LG Mennonites. We have paid less attention to their religious beliefs and practices, especially as they relate to health and illness. The purpose of my research program was to address this void. It has been a journey that, of necessity, required the development not only of particular ways of performing the research itself but of relaying the findings to the LG Mennonites and those who care for them. This process would not have been possible without the dedication of the research advisory committee members who worked with me on the various studies. Of equal importance, the studies could not have succeeded had the LG Mennonites whom we interviewed not expressed interest in our work and agreed to take the risks associated with participating in it. The research assistants were also an integral part of the process, given their abilities not only to speak Plautdietsch (Low German) but also to gently encourage interviewees to express their views.

The focus of this book is the LG Mennonites, and it serves as an example of how to work respectfully and effectively with a minority religious group. Cultural competence is key to developing and implementing care that considers a client's attitudes, beliefs, and customs in relation to religious diversity. This process is applicable to other similar groups, and I hope it will be examined and applied in that light.

ACKNOWLEDGMENTS

Preparing this book has been a journey of excitement, anticipation, and fulfillment. It would never have been written without the involvement and support of a number of people. I am grateful to the Low German Mennonites whom I met throughout the years, including the many who agreed to be interviewed and to talk about their lives, knowledge, and beliefs. I thank the research advisory committee members, whose dedication to understanding LG Mennonites and to sharing that knowledge with me helped ensure the successful completion of the projects. Mennonite Central Committee Canada was very helpful, particularly John Janzen, former Low German coordinator, as were Dave and Margaret Penner, who hosted me during my visit to Durango Colony, Mexico. The research assistants in the various projects not only collected data but shared their perspectives about a number of topics related to what is discussed here. The final two projects were coordinated by HaiYan Fan, whose attention to detail, insights, and pure joy at being in the field made for interesting conversations but also some fun in exploring and learning together about Mennonite communities. My thanks also go to the undergraduate research assistants who worked on the projects and to the numerous family members, friends, and colleagues who cheered me on from the sidelines. I would like to thank the clinical agencies with which I worked: Alberta Health Services, Southern Health–Santé Sud and

Eden Health Care Services in Manitoba, and the Canadian Mental Health Association in Elgin, Ontario. One other clinical agency that provided generous support for the research was Salem Home in Winkler, Manitoba. Their support in all phases of the research projects is truly appreciated.

I will always be grateful to Mary Walters, who provided professional editorial guidance and expertise throughout all stages of the book. I appreciate the support and interest of Darcy Cullen at UBC Press, who ensured that this book came to fruition, and the feedback from the peer reviewers, which helped to shape and strengthen it.

I would like to acknowledge the following funding that supported the research discussed here: Alberta Heritage Foundation for Medical Research, which funded Kanadier Mennonites' Health and Illness, and Canadian Institutes of Health Research, which funded Exploring Kanadier Mennonite Women's Health: Identifying Their Knowledge and Need for Health Promotion, The Discovery of Death and Dying Beliefs among Low German Speaking Mennonites: Application to Best Practice Guidelines, and Mental Health Wellness and Illness Knowledge and Beliefs among Low German-Speaking Mennonites: Development of Best Practice Guidelines. Funding for this book was provided directly from grants for the last two projects.

CARING FOR THE LOW GERMAN MENNONITES

INTRODUCTION

Canadians often reflect with pride upon their Multiculturalism Act, which became federal law in 1988; most believe that it allows Canada to address its societal changes in ways that other countries cannot match. According to some policy experts, this act has historically dealt with only two components of our cultural makeup – ethnicity and race – although there are now calls to formally recognize religious diversity as a third area of focus (Kunz, 2009; Fadden & Townsend, 2009).

Until recently, clear discourse about religious diversity in Canada has been lacking, including how governments and other institutions address it (Fadden & Townsend, 2009). We tend to focus on the religious perspectives of new immigrants and refugees, especially those who are not Roman Catholics or Anglicans, Canada's traditional Christian denominations (Kunz, 2009). Muslim immigrants and refugees entering Canada have received particular attention of late (Kunz, 2009). And though we most certainly do need to understand the beliefs and world views of new arrivals, we sometimes fail to recognize and understand those of minority religious groups who have lived in Canada for many years.

This book aims to advance conversation in Canada about the importance of recognizing and understanding religious diversity in providing appropriate and equitable health care to all individuals and communities. This discussion is based in over twenty years of work with a unique religious population, the Low German (LG) Mennonites.

This book has a twofold purpose. First, it underscores the fact that health providers must consider and assess religious diversity if they wish to fully understand their clients. It is essential to remember that religious diversity is not synonymous with cultural diversity; having a strong religious faith is not the same as adhering to cultural beliefs and practices. In this book, "religion" refers to institutionalized beliefs and practices, and is viewed as a subset of culture (Pesut, Fowler, Taylor, Reimer-Kirkham, & Sawatzky, 2008). It is based in the conviction that a higher power exists and that it is linked with one's life course – including such essential elements as whether one becomes ill and when one dies (Anderson, 1990, cited in Hickman, 2006). In contrast, cultural beliefs and practices are generally less spiritually significant and can incorporate a comprehensive range of behaviours that relate to activities such as wedding ceremonies or the celebration of specific events (such as Thanksgiving Day); they may also involve beliefs such as the idea that certain foods have healing properties (Newman Giger, 2012). Although cultural beliefs and practices usually exist in conjunction with religious perspectives, in most cases they form only one element of the larger sociocultural religious context. My research with LG Mennonites revealed that religion was the primary determining factor in all their everyday activities. In most cases, their belief in God was so deeply rooted and strictly adhered to that they went far beyond merely observing tradition. As a result, they shared certain views about health and illness, and whether and how to use health services.

The second underlying contention of this book is that because religion is so important for some individuals, cultural competence is an essential aspect of acute, community-based, or other kinds of care. Educators who work in the health care professions must introduce their students to cultural competence and teach them about its applicability in providing care for diverse clients. Health care organizations must enable their staff to access continuing education that instructs them about the religious beliefs and practices of the clients in their geographic area and includes meeting the expectation of cultural competence when providing care. In addition, they need to create policies to guarantee that religious diversity is addressed during the assessment, implementation, and evaluation of care.

Cultural Competence: An Essential Part of Health Care

Providing care to ethnically, culturally, or religiously diverse groups can be both challenging and rewarding. It requires understanding, acknowledging, and working with individuals whose ideas differ from those of mainstream culture. Over the years, there has been considerable discussion in the health care field about the need to address our increasingly diverse society (Erlen, 1998; Wood & Schwass, 1993) through the application of concepts such as cultural awareness, cultural sensitivity, and cultural competence (Wepa, 2003).

Cultural awareness is defined as understanding the ways in which culture forms an individual's beliefs and values (De & Richardson, 2008), whereas cultural sensitivity refers to respecting, valuing, and understanding other cultures while also being aware of one's own (Erlen, 1998). It extends from cultural awareness, asking health professionals to develop their knowledge and change their behaviour to recognize the power differentials between groups, as well as their historical and social roots (Polaschek, 1998). Cultural sensitivity increases one's understanding of how cultures affect both personal and professional identities. Without it, cultural interaction will be ineffective (Narayanasamy & White, 2005); when health care providers demonstrate respect for cultural differences, they are more likely to provide impartial care (Erlen, 1998).

Cultural competence flows naturally from cultural awareness and sensitivity, a point "on a continuum of cultural approaches" (Brascoupe & Waters, 2009, p. 10). It has three components: awareness, knowledge, and skills (Alizadeh & Chavan, 2016). That is, it consists of the culture-related awareness, knowledge, and skills that are necessary to provide effective care to diverse groups, and it exists at both the individual and the organizational levels (Dreachslin, Gilbert, & Malone, 2013). In this book, I focus predominantly on the individual level and define cultural competence as a process through which knowledge and skills in relation to a client's attitudes, beliefs, and customs are developed and applied in the provision of care (Parisa, Reza, Afsaneh, & Sarieh, 2016). In the health care setting, such competence leads to effectively addressing the cultural context of the client (Campinha-Bacote, 2002).

Cultural competence is also an important aspect of addressing the health care disparities and social justice issues that arise from inequitable life circumstances among diverse groups (Alizadeh & Chavan, 2016; Dreachslin et al., 2013; Lehman, Fenza, & Hollinger-Smith, 2012; Shen, 2015). It is a way to focus on patient-centred care to allow for collaboration and active participation of patients and their family members (Dreachslin et al., 2013). To achieve this and to acknowledge the multicultural context within which care occurs, providers must work from a stance of reflective practice that is based in critical thinking (Blanchet Garneau, 2016). Working this way can lead to improved clinical care. It also enables providers to consider the social and political structures that can impede the delivery and uptake of care among diverse groups.

The Cultural Competence Development Model

The Cultural Competence Development Model (Blanchet Garneau, 2013; Blanchet Garneau & Pepin, 2015) is a valuable tool for health care providers who work in a variety of culturally diverse settings. It can also be used when religion and beliefs are the main aspect of diversity. This model is based on defining cultural competence as "a complex know-act grounded in critical reflection and action, which the health care professional draws upon to provide culturally safe, congruent, and effective care in partnership with individuals, families, and communities living health experiences, and which takes into account the social and political dimensions of care" (Blanchet Garneau & Pepin, 2015, p. 12). This definition reflects a constructivist perspective, which emphasizes multiple, socially constructed realities (Blanchet Garneau & Pepin, 2015) while recognizing that power relations exist and influence one's reality (Guba & Lincoln, 1994, 2005, cited in Blanchet Garneau & Pepin, 2015). Cultural competence is both dynamic and complex but variable according to the social context. It is a "process of reflection and action" (Blanchet Garneau & Pepin, 2015, p. 13) that can lead to the development of new knowledge of providing culturally congruent care.

The Cultural Competence Development Model consists of three levels (Blanchet Garneau, 2013). The first of these, being open to the differing realities of practice, encompasses

- forging a relationship with patients by showing openness to their beliefs and ideas while also emphasizing the importance of communication
- working outside usual practice by building awareness of structural limitations and the care challenges in culturally diverse contexts
- reinventing one's practice in action by acknowledging the gap between theory and practice, and by employing approaches used by one's more experienced colleagues.

The second level, challenging one's practice in a culturally diverse context, involves

- building a relationship with a patient by looking for commonalities between oneself and that person, focusing on the patient, and using a variety of communication strategies
- working outside usual practice by taking the patient's environment into account when care is being provided, and by working within the structural limitations
- reinventing one's practice in action by taking the risk of changing one's own model.

The third level, integrating the realities of practice within the culturally diverse context, comprises

- building a relationship with the patient by incorporating differences, establishing a partnership, and communicating with discernment
- working outside the usual practice framework, which includes circumventing structural limitations and considering the patient and the provider as core components of a dynamic system
- reinventing one's practice by acting at the right moment and integrating one's model into practice.

Health care providers who apply this model may discover that their current practice does not meet client needs and may come to question and modify their approach. This can occur only if they develop authentic relationships with clients and realize that gaps exist between current theory and practice. It is essential for providers to think critically and to reflect on their practice, acknowledging the diverse environment in which they work. Applying the Cultural Competence Development Model has a dual benefit: it can correct the inaccurate ideas of practitioners regarding religiously diverse groups, and it can aid them in rectifying patients' faulty perceptions of health and illness, thus producing a positive outcome for everyone involved.

Working with Low German Mennonites

Low German Mennonites began to arrive in Canada during the 1870s. Their communities are concentrated primarily in southern Alberta, Saskatchewan, Manitoba, Ontario, and Nova Scotia, with a total population of approximately 100,000. They retain a community-focused lifestyle that dictates their choice of clothing, education, employment, and social interactions, and they purposefully separate themselves from the outside world. They speak a Low German dialect known as Mennonite Plautdietsch (Cox, 2008; Hedges, 1996). Only the church leaders (that is, male leaders) typically use Literary Dutch or High German and then only on formal occasions, such as at church services, funerals, and weddings (Sawatzky, 2005). The English-language skills of community members may be imperfect; women, in particular, have more limited exposure to English. LG Mennonites belong to a range of churches, from conservative to liberal, and their beliefs and practices vary both within and across congregations. For example, some conservative LG Mennonites do not use technological devices such as computers, whereas others – though still conservative – use them if they are of benefit to the community. More liberal LG Mennonites may use such gadgets as often as mainstream Canadians. All LG Mennonites rely on the Bible as the primary source of truth and guidance for their decisions and lifestyle choices. They have traditionally been, and continue to be, primarily involved in agricultural work and have greatly contributed to the dynamic nature of rural Canada.

Since 1995, I have learned many lessons from my various community development and research projects with LG Mennonites. The program has required an ongoing commitment to winning and maintaining the trust of this unique, diverse religious group.[1]

My first contact as a researcher with the LG Mennonite community was in 1995, when I supervised undergraduate nursing students in a senior community health course as they carried out cultural-assessment interviews in southern Alberta. To assist them, I conducted the first interview with an LG Mennonite couple and, concealing their identity, shared the transcript with the class to show how I had proceeded. When the project ended, I reviewed all forty-four interviews and prepared a final report for a local health unit (Kulig, 1995).[2] With one of the students, I also wrote an article based on the interviews to highlight the health needs of LG Mennonites in southern Alberta (Kulig & McCaslin, 1998).

Following that experience, I helped found the Southern Alberta Kanadier Association (SAKA), an umbrella group that represents health, education, and community personnel to address the needs of LG Mennonites. Through SAKA and my contacts with the health region,

I worked with undergraduate nursing students for several years as they created and implemented community development projects with LG Mennonites, such as health fairs, anatomy and physiology classes for women, and babysitting courses for Mennonite girls (accompanied by their mothers as observers). I helped students generate the projects and attended their presentations wherever and whenever they occurred throughout southern Alberta. The LG Mennonites displayed a great thirst for knowledge and were enthusiastic about what they learned. I particularly remember their interest and keenness when the students demonstrated anatomy and physiology using pig hearts, which have a remarkable likeness to human hearts. The women were also fascinated by a project in which they washed their hands and then applied a special substance to their hands. It would glow under ultraviolet light if they'd done a less than thorough job; the glow represented the bacteria that had not been washed off.

In subsequent years, I engaged in a wide range of activities relating to LG Mennonites. In 2001, the Chinook Regional Health Authority asked me to evaluate the work of the health promotion specialist who was responsible for the LG Mennonites in southwestern Alberta; later renamed the LG Mennonite liaison worker, this person provided translation at health care facilities, arranged for families to attend specialist appointments, and educated parents about health conditions such as genetic disorders and diabetes. My evaluation included interviewing LG Mennonite families whom the specialist had assisted to determine their satisfaction and generate any recommendations to the health region. The specialist ensured that the regional health authority increasingly took into account the LG Mennonites' own health priorities in delivering care to the community.

In my capacity as a researcher, I also interviewed LG Mennonite women about nutrition and food issues (Johnston et al., 1997). Because I did not wish to use a tape recorder, I worked with a woman who spoke Plautdietsch. As she translated each of my interview questions and the responses to them, I made brief notes that I later transcribed more fully.

Throughout such activities, I visited homeschool sites and other facilities used by LG Mennonites and was a guest in their homes. I learned about where they lived and had previously lived, their living conditions, their degree of isolation, their family networks and support systems, and how they interacted with each other. I learned, for example, that the links between individuals formed the essential basis for social relationships and connections within the community.

After I had worked on these various projects, I presented the possibility of conducting additional research in the community SAKA members and respected Mennonites. This led to a more extensive research program than I had imagined. Since then, I have conducted four studies with LG Mennonites to generate information about their perspectives on four issues: health and illness (2000–02); women's health and sexuality (2003–08); death and dying (2009–14); and mental health (2012–16).[3] All the research received ethical clearance from my institution and from the relevant clinical agencies in the provinces where it was conducted.[4]

Some authors contend that researchers must determine whether their projects are morally justified (Liamputtong, 2010). The goal of my research – to help LG Mennonites receive appropriate health care – served as a solid rationale for our studies. Given the desire of LG Mennonites to remain separate from the world, and my opportunity to generate information with them about their health perspectives, I believe that it was morally appropriate for me to act as a conduit for their voices and to share their views in a manner that complemented their ethical and religious beliefs.

During my presentations in all three of the provinces where I performed the research and elsewhere, LG Mennonite and other Mennonite groups responded positively, confirming that my information and portrayal of the community were sound. In one case, when I was presenting via webinar to the Kansas State Farmworkers group, the LG Mennonite liaison worker there commented that my presentation reflected her own upbringing in Mexico. Throughout the years, I have been contacted by nurses with Mennonite backgrounds who worked with this population via the Mennonite Central Committee (MCC), a nongovernmental organization with offices in Mexico, and they have endorsed my findings and observations.

All my research studies followed the same process. The investigation was planned and implemented with the full cooperation of an advisory group.[5] Trained research assistants (RAs) interviewed LG Mennonite individuals and sometimes couples.[6] To avoid offending respondents, some of whom believed that the use of technology did not align with their religious values, interviews were not recorded. Instead, a summary – including exact wording and Plautdietsch words on specific ideas and topics – was used to highlight their sentiments.[7] Subsequently, the RA prepared a transcript, which I then checked. I spoke with the RA over the telephone or in person, providing feedback to use in future interviews and seeking clarification about the transcripts when required. In all the studies, our data analysis was conducted in a similar manner. I read the transcripts and field notes many times to identify themes that illustrated the views of participants (Braun & Clarke, 2006; Liamputtong, 2013).[8]

I also conducted fieldwork among LG Mennonites in Belize, Mexico, and Canada. In 2003, through discussions with two local health committees in Belize, I arranged for two nursing students to carry out their senior practicums in the LG Mennonite communities of Blue Creek and Spanish Lookout. In both locales, the health committee consisted of three couples who oversaw the management of services, including organizing and staffing clinics and providing other services, such as ambulances. The committee agreed that the students could come to Blue Creek and Spanish Lookout for their practicums. My fieldwork focused on observing interactions between individuals and at events and gatherings, as well as talking with people about their roles. For example, I observed male and female dress, acceptable types of transportation, and what women and men did at community functions.

In 2010, I attended an MCC biannual networking meeting in Cuauhtémoc, Mexico, with the local Mennonite liaison worker and

LingLing Fan, who was the project coordinator for the study on death and dying that was under way at the time.[9] We stayed at the Steinreich Bible College and toured the local *Altenheim* (senior residents' home); *Huffungsheim* (home for people with disabilities, including those with mental health or other problems such as fetal alcohol spectrum disorder); *Friedensplatz* (orphanage and safe house for vulnerable children); schools (different ones for children from conservative and liberal churches); and the substance abuse centre, Centro de Rehabilitación Luz en mi Camino (Light My Way Rehabilitation Centre). We also attended choir evenings and Sunday service at Mennonite churches. I drove through the villages, noting their geographical differences, and visited local cheese factories. At the MCC meeting, we presented our preliminary findings from the study on death and dying. We received valuable feedback, which was later incorporated into the revisions, and made contacts with conference delegates from Ontario who would prove invaluable for the subsequent study on mental health and wellness.

In 2012, I visited the MCC office in Durango Colony, Mexico, for eight days. I interviewed women and men in the community, attended a funeral and church services, went to a *pharmacia* (pharmacy) and clinic run by an LG Mennonite woman, and visited a bone-setter (an LG Mennonite who diagnoses and treats a variety of ailments).

In 2013, LingLing Fan and I went to La Crete, Alberta, an isolated community that was established during the 1950s and includes a variety of Mennonite groups. Some of its members had immigrated from Bolivia. During our time there, we met with local health providers, most of whom had a Mennonite background, regarding our research.

Although this book focuses on the lives of Low German Mennonites in Canada, participants who had resided in other countries, such as Mexico or Belize, were asked to speak about their time there. When relevant, their views about life in these countries are also discussed here.

By combining what we observed in homes and at community events, learned in discussions with our advisory groups, and heard in our interviews, we compiled a robust body of knowledge not only about this group's ideas concerning health and illness, but also about a range of other topics. By and large, participants had had little opportunity to think about their beliefs or to talk to others about their perspectives, a fact that was especially true for members of the most conservative churches. As a result, the interviews became an empowering experience for many of them.

It is important to note that, according to the Mennonite members of our advisory group, the experience also posed a potential threat to the authority of LG Mennonite ministers. For example, we heard that the clergymen were concerned about the interviews, probably because they encouraged participants to reflect on their own beliefs and practices as well as those of the church. Such reflection is not encouraged in conservative churches. Throughout all our research studies, a number of respondents initially proved reluctant to speak and found it difficult to discuss their beliefs in detail. In part, they were apprehensive about providing the right answers, but this fear gradually diminished as the RA reassured them that whatever they said would be the right answer. By the end of the interviews, they often made comments such as, "I had never given these ideas any thought!" and "I have lots to think about now." Even when they were willing to express their opinions, not all of them – both males and females – could provide details in every instance. We assumed that this arose from feeling uncomfortable with our questions or, more importantly, from never having considered them before.

During my early years of working with LG Mennonites, including my first research studies in Alberta, I attended community events whenever possible. I typically learned about the event from an LG Mennonite woman, who assured me that I was welcome to come. Few non-LG Mennonites attended, so having a contact was helpful; she introduced me to her circle of friends, which enhanced my comfort. Sometimes, I attended concerts given by visiting choirs, usually from Manitoba; these were held in a community hall after Sunday services and might include a shared meal at the end of the performance. While the audience waited for the singing to start, it was common to see older women sitting together in the back, eating sunflower seeds and spitting the husks into ice cream buckets on the floor. Children played outside or in the hall, and groups of people – separated by gender – chatted, the pitch of Plautdietsch rising with excitement and emphasis.

The women and men to whom I was introduced showed quiet curiosity about who I was and why I was there. Some posed very blunt questions, asking if I was married (when I first began research with this group, I was not married; after I did marry, I said so and explained that my husband had two sons from a previous marriage). When asked what church I attended, I replied that I went to no church at the moment. Some people merely looked at me, often paying particular attention to my clothing. Others wanted to know if I was a Mennonite, if I had attended singing events before, and whether I worked. After answering such questions, I reciprocated by asking the women where they lived, where their husbands worked, and where they had been born.

Typically, the women with whom I became acquainted had not progressed beyond Grade 4 in school and did not work outside the home. I had, and did. To add to the distance between us, I did not work for any formal agency with which they were familiar, such as the local MCC office or the public education system. My explanation that I was a nurse who taught at the university and did not work as a clinician was not entirely helpful. They reacted positively to my nursing background, and they understood that nursing students needed to be taught. But they did not comprehend why I was interested in *them*. Conscious of choosing my words carefully, I explained that nurses, physicians, and other providers needed to know more about them to give them the best care possible. I would gather the necessary information during my conversations with members of their group, and it would help health professionals to provide care. The question of why I was spending time with LG Mennonites and why I wanted to know about them was repeatedly raised during the years that I conducted this research. Whenever it was voiced by any LG Mennonite or stakeholder who worked with the group, I gave similar explanations to those outlined above, hoping to reduce apprehension about my presence and my questions.

Throughout the research, I observed relationships within the LG Mennonite communities and with non-LG Mennonites such as myself. I noticed a number of differences between and within the groups, and that what was said to be happening sometimes contradicted what was actually happening. For instance, no group condoned alcohol consumption among its members, but some individuals did drink (of all ages and both genders), and some were alcoholics. Because of the general denial that alcohol was being used, support was often lacking for people who were struggling to make positive changes in their lives.

Occasionally, I encountered practices that were not compatible with my own beliefs in fairness and social justice. One example was in the treatment of women. Some groups purposefully blamed women for the ill treatment they received from their spouse, claiming that they deserved it. Upon further examination, I found that women's opinions and ideas were not always acknowledged or considered and that they were expected to acquiesce when told what to do. I had experienced similar issues when I worked with other diverse groups, where I had learned that I was not responsible for making changes among them and that I simply needed to accept certain circumstances and situations. I realized that change would arise naturally once the group came in contact with the values and beliefs of the society around it, probably initiated by its younger members (who were exposed to education and opportunities outside their community) and by those who were already questioning its values, beliefs, and behaviours. I learned not to feel responsible for the changes that would occur but to recognize that exposure to outsiders – myself and others – would be part of the process and that change is inevitable for all groups. I was also able to reflect on my own cultural background and to perceive that my family was not exempt from this process. My maternal and paternal grandparents came from Poland and raised their children in Canada; as a grandchild, I witnessed how their lives had changed and realized that such changes facilitated integration into the larger society. As aunts and uncles married non-Polish people, diet and customs were naturally modified. This did not mean that Polish customs and values were abandoned, but rather that certain lifestyle behaviours were invariably altered as needed.

Throughout my experiences with LG Mennonites and my exposure to the differences between group members, I benefitted from discussions with the research team – particularly those who came from a Mennonite background. Within the research project, we did what we could to help individuals obtain appropriate assistance for challenging family circumstances or when they needed care for complex conditions. For example, I made referrals to the LG Mennonite liaison worker, who followed up with women and their families and provided support and services as required. I also found that I needed to accept some situations, as I did not have the power to change them. However, when I felt that the legal rights of individuals were being violated, I was professionally obligated to inform human services personnel.

Applying the Cultural Competence Model in LG Mennonite Communities

For LG Mennonites, religion is central to all aspects of life. It dictates everything from their choice of clothing to their social interactions. Their practices and behaviours were originally developed to maintain their separation from the outside world but have also produced misunderstandings between themselves and others. Non-Mennonites who have attempted to provide them with care have not been immune to this problem, and the failure in communication has revealed that we need to find more appropriate ways of working collaboratively with this group. Our use of cultural competence in developing collaborative care with LG Mennonites helped us to identify connections between their religious perspectives and the unique factors that place them at risk for health disparities. This work was intended to engender positive outcomes for LG Mennonites by providing guidelines that would enable an engaged and enlightened provider to apply sound principles. The ultimate goal is better health among LG Mennonites and, through the involvement of the community itself, a greater awareness of their care options. This book is a case example of cultural competence in action.

The religious beliefs of LG Mennonites influence the values they associate with wellness and well-being, their understanding of health and illness, and their decisions regarding health behaviours and whether to seek care. For example, they see good hygiene and cleanliness as extremely important. Thus, when a new mother lacks the energy to clean her home because she suffers from postpartum depression, she and her family are frequently perceived as lazy. The people who are responsible for making decisions about her health – including her husband and her minister – commonly do not realize that her listlessness is a sign of depression. Rather than obtaining support for her or helping with the housework themselves, they are likely to exhort her to pray and to apply herself. A health practitioner who has developed cultural competence with the community will understand this context and can help the woman receive the care she needs.

When working with LG Mennonites, caregivers need to remember that ideas about health matters will vary depending on which church their patients attend. Conservative LG Mennonites generally feel that they must remain separate from the mainstream, and their health-related decisions will reflect this conviction. Members of more liberal churches are more likely to accept care that requires interaction with outsiders.

Clergymen play a vital role in the daily lives of LG Mennonites, a fact that culturally competent care must take into account. Parishioners must consult with their ministers regarding care plans, and ministers must agree to the administration of treatments such as medication and counselling. Practitioners need to recognize that clients who reject a recommended treatment plan may do so because they or their minister feel that it does not accord with the tenets of the faith. It is always important for practitioners to acknowledge and respectfully inquire about a client's beliefs, so that they can be taken into consideration when planning and providing care; this helps to satisfy both client and family that all their needs are being met.

The lessons from the case study shared in this book can be applied by clinicians, researchers, and policy makers who work with, or are responsible for attending to the needs of, groups that live on the margins of society due to their religious beliefs. By engaging in discussions related to the issues covered here, we can achieve a better understanding of the diversity of our society as a whole and of the unique perspectives of its individual groups. The end result is not only further understanding of health care consumers and improvements to research skills, but also the development of public policy that will help provide equitable care to all citizens, regardless of their religious or cultural identity.

1

A BRIEF HISTORY OF THE LOW GERMAN MENNONITES

The history of Low German Mennonite migration is characterized by the group's determination to remain true to its beliefs. Since the sixteenth century, LG Mennonites have migrated frequently – within Europe, from Europe to North America, and then throughout North and South America – to find locations where they can exercise religious and educational autonomy, remaining isolated from external influences. The migrations have always occurred in reaction to political, religious, and economic issues (Driedger, 2000).

Low German Mennonites find their roots in the Anabaptist movement, which began in 1521 in Germany as part of the Protestant Reformation (Friesen, 2011). Anabaptists believe that baptism must be conducted in adulthood, when believers are mature enough to make reasoned decisions about religious matters. In 1536, Menno Simons, a Catholic priest in the Netherlands, left his church and became a leader in the Dutch Anabaptist movement; his followers became known as Mennonites (Driedger, 2000; Friesen, 2011). He believed that Christian faith should be grounded in the Bible, that the church was central to all aspects of life, and that non-resistance and pacifism were necessary values. For Mennonites, being a Christian entailed sharing both spiritually and physically with fellow believers; having a visible or organized church made them responsible to one another in practical ways.

Migration History

In Europe, Mennonites were persecuted for their beliefs, and governments imposed limitations on their lifestyle. As a result, they began to move from one country to another, seeking a place where they could honour their religious principles. In the late eighteenth century, Catherine II of Russia issued a manifesto inviting Europeans to settle in her country, and Mennonites in Prussia responded (Friesen, 2011). Between 1788 and 1830, thousands arrived in southern Russia (Ukraine or New Russia), establishing the settlements of Chortitza and Molotschna (Dyck, 1967; Friesen, 2011; Krahn & Sawatzky, 1990). In 1800, Czar Paul I, Catherine's son, signed a hundred-year "Privilegium," which assured the Mennonites that they could practise their religion, maintain their own schools, and be exempt from military service – thereby indicating Russia's willingness to respect their pacifism (Friesen, 2011).

Initially, the move to Russia worked well for the Mennonites; however, by 1870, the government had passed a ruling that required colonists to serve in the military. Meanwhile, a Mennonite delegation had travelled to North America to explore the possibility of migrating there; the threat of losing this population spurred the Russian government to reconsider its ultimatum. Negotiations ensued, with the result that the Mennonites were offered an alternative to military service: compulsory forestry service. However, a number of them saw this option as unacceptable because they would still be in service to the government, and they continued to pursue the idea of relocating to North America. Interest in migration was fuelled by the discomfort of conservative Mennonites regarding social and political developments that were occurring in New Russia, such as proposed changes to education that would lead to an expanded liberal arts curriculum. They felt that the innovations did not respect their principles or way of life, and they saw flight as the most appropriate solution to the problem (Friesen, 2011).

After negotiations with the US and Canadian governments, which reassured the Mennonites that they would be exempt from military service and that their religious and educational autonomy would be protected, many moved to the United States and Canada, commencing in the 1870s (Friesen, 2011). Some authors agree that those who left Russia were the more conservative European Mennonites and refer to them as Old Colony to signify that they came from the first or oldest colony in Russia (Quiring, 1997). Estimates vary regarding the number of migrants but are generally around seventeen to eighteen thousand (Friesen, 2011; Loewen, 2001). According to Friesen (2011), seven thousand moved to Manitoba and ten thousand to the United States.

In Manitoba, the Mennonites originally settled on the east side of the Red River, in an area referred to as the East Reserve. In Russia, they had designed their communities according to a German system called *Strassendorf*,[1] in which houses line a central street and the farmsteads extend behind them. The East Reserve land was deemed unsuitable for laying out villages in the Strassendorf manner, so some people moved to the west side of the Red River, to the West Reserve – near modern-day Winkler and Morden – as it was better suited to their preferred village design (Friesen, 2011).

Mennonite village life in Manitoba was based upon the values of mutual support and brotherhood, rather than on conforming to state-imposed laws. The Mennonites who settled in Manitoba came as groups from Russia and did not disperse, in part to maintain their religious principles. They also replicated their community structure, which included the administration of the village, ensuring that civil life conformed to their beliefs. For example, the villages in Manitoba elected members of the Waisenamt, an institution within the village government that cared for orphans, widows, and widowers (Friesen, 2011). A combination of three key elements – an agricultural lifestyle, a religious and civil structure, and a fostering of equality and mutual support – meant that the Mennonites could retain their isolation, self-sufficiency, and distinctive interpretations of the word of God.

The Mennonites also migrated within Canada. As early as 1895, approximately one thousand moved from Manitoba to the Hague and Osler areas of Saskatchewan, and an additional nine hundred moved to the region of Swift Current, Saskatchewan, in 1905 (Quiring, 1997). They also settled in southern Alberta at the turn of the century but never established a Strassendorf form of village life.

Despite their hopes for long-term harmony in Manitoba, the Mennonites began to feel that their communities and lifestyle were under threat from various external influences. One of these originated in the United States. Unlike in Canada, where Mennonites had maintained their cohesion in villages, those who relocated to America had scattered and begun to make fundamental changes to their lives. As early as 1883, Mennonite missionaries from the United States began to proselytize in Manitoba, encouraging its Mennonite inhabitants to change their village structure and convert to a new church. Some individuals did accept their guidance, making such drastic changes that they had to withdraw from their village lives, including the organizations to which they belonged. Others felt that the Christianity of the American missionaries was narrow and – importantly – less Biblical than their own, with a focus on the individual rather than the communal way of life. Conflicts began to arise in the Mennonite villages of Manitoba (Friesen, 2011).

A number of Mennonites were becoming disaffected with wider Canadian society. Although the agreements with the federal government were grounded in good intentions on both sides, once the First World War began, the public began to resent the Mennonites due to their opposition to military service (Friesen, 2011). However, the issue that caused the most concern for the Mennonites themselves was the passing of Manitoba's School Attendance Act in March 1916, which decreed that all children must attend public school and that the language of instruction would be English (Friesen, 2011; Loewen, 2013). Hence, in 1916, the LG Mennonites became subject to taxes and fines because their children were not attending school (Friesen, 2011). In some cases, they were jailed for refusing to send their children to school (Quiring, 1997). Following the First World War, Ottawa responded to widespread disapproval of pacifism by refusing to admit pacifist immigrants, including the Mennonites, Hutterites, and Doukhobors (Friesen, 2011). Once again, the most conservative Mennonites considered relocating, hoping to find a safe haven that would assure their religious, educational, and linguistic freedom (Castro, 2004).

Old Colony Mennonite delegates travelled to Mexico and Paraguay, where they negotiated with the respective governments in pursuit of terms that would protect their way of life after they migrated. The negotiations were a success: they would control their own schools, where lessons would be taught in German and based on church principles; they would be exempt from military service; and they would not be barred from purchasing land in the future (Loewen, 2013).

In March 1922, the first chartered trains containing six thousand Old Colony and Sommerfelder Mennonites left Plum Coulee, Manitoba, and Swift Current, heading for Mexico. (Sommerfelder is a less conservative branch of the Mennonite Church than Old Colony, but not liberal.) They made their way to the Bustillos Valley in the northern state of Chihuahua and farther south to the Guatimapé Valley in Durango State (Loewen, 2013; Quiring, 1997). They set up their villages according to the Strassendorf style, just as they had for centuries (Quiring, 1997). Each village had a semi-autonomous civic structure, and schooling, justice, and agricultural planning were regulated by an internal governing body (Friesen, 2011). In the Bustillos Valley near Cuauhtémoc, Chihuahua, the villages were aptly named Manitoba and Swift Current Colonies. They usually had German names as well but were referred to in Spanish as "Campo" and were assigned a number so that Mexican authorities and local people could easily find them (Quiring, 1997). There are now more than forty-five villages in the Cuauhtémoc area of Chihuahua State and fifty-eight in Durango State.

In 1926, a group of Mennonites migrated from Canada to Chaco, Paraguay (Loewen, 2013). Others relocated from Mexico to Paraguay, and another group moved from Canada to Paraguay in 1948. In 1956, some Mennonite settlers emigrated from Chaco to Santa Cruz, Bolivia; several more colonies were established in this region during the 1960s, when Mennonites from Mexico moved there to maintain their conservative lifestyle. Others from northern Alberta joined these groups in Santa Cruz during the 1970s.

In 1958, approximately five thousand Mennonites left Chihuahua and arrived in Belize (Dyck, 1967; Pauls, 2004). Some had decided to leave Mexico due to its newly formed social security program, which they feared jeopardized the exemptions they received from the government. The new program would determine benefits based on contributions, which the Mennonites would not pay. In addition, the newly instituted mandatory national registration program was a negative reminder of a similar national registry that had been implemented in Canada before the First World War. The registration would require the Mennonites to be photographed – a concern, given their non-acceptance of graven images (Loewen, 2013). Following the move to Belize, some eventually moved on again: concerned about security and safety, a small group left Belize in 1984 and established Northfield Settlement in Nova Scotia (Pauls, 2004).

Remaining in and Returning to Canada

What of the Mennonites who chose to remain in Canada while their co-religionists set off for Mexico? They were comfortable with the changes in their adopted country, and staying gave them access to extra land as their fellow community members vacated their properties (Quiring, 1997). They also accepted public education and engaged in employment that was not agricultural. Eventually, they experienced an evangelical movement. Evangelical Mennonites believe that once they are converted, their salvation is assured, whereas conservative Mennonites feel that they cannot be assured salvation even if they never deviate from the word of God (Guenther, 2004; Loewen, 2013). The evangelical movement also emphasizes that individuals should study the Bible for themselves rather than depending on the minister for its interpretation (Guenther, 2004). The decision of some families to remain in Canada led to differences in opinion among relatives and often produced lengthy separations between them. In some instances, the discrepancies in belief were so great that family members severed their connections (Loewen, 2013; Quiring, 1997).

During my 2010 trip to Cuauhtémoc, I met two LG Mennonite cousins. The family of one had stayed in Canada, whereas the other family had migrated to Mexico. As a result of this, the cousins' fathers, who were siblings, spent their lives in two different countries. The Canadian-based brother and his descendants had been exposed to a range of changes and opportunities that were not available to the brother in Mexico. It was interesting to compare the two cousins and to see the stark contrast in how they dressed, what they did for a living, how they lived, and the degree of conservatism of their religious beliefs.

Not all the Mennonites who journeyed to Mexico decided to remain there. Many shuttled between Mexico and Canada. Some returned to Canada during the mid-1930s when drought struck Chihuahua and Durango, and farming became untenable (Loewen, 2013; Quiring, 1997); they also left in response to a threat from the Mexican government to close their schools (Loewen, 2013). Although the threat never materialized, some had already chosen to return to Canada (Loewen, 2013). Another factor that influenced their return was the ease with which they could cross the US-Canada border. Because many were eligible for Canadian citizenship and benefitted from favourable immigration policies, they could migrate strategically, improving their standard of living while simultaneously escaping population pressures, landlessness, and religious strife (Quiring, 1997).

Droughts in Mexico fuelled further migration back to Canada. In the 1950s and 1960s, LG Mennonites travelled from Mexico to Ontario for agricultural jobs, hoping to alleviate the poverty they experienced at home; as families, they worked wherever crops such as potatoes and tomatoes required hand picking. Some returned to the familiar landscape of Manitoba, where they could engage in similar farming occupations (Quiring, 1997). Some tell stories of the discrimination that returnees encountered from Mennonites who had remained in Canada; living and working conditions were not always ideal. Over time, some LG Mennonites from Mexico decided to remain in Canada and others continued to join them. From the 1950s to the 1970s, over eight thousand had moved to Ontario, while others relocated to the second destination of choice –Manitoba. The migration to Alberta started in earnest with approximately three thousand Mennonites migrating to that province by 1993 (Quiring, 1997). Those who stayed in Mexico often criticized them for returning to a country that had betrayed them. Regardless of their provincial destination, all experienced a break with the traditional teachings of the conservative churches (Old Colony and Sommerfelder) in Mexico. Those who returned to Canada after the Second World War found that it offered a variety of social programs to aid migrants, but there were negatives as well. For many, the move north meant reducing ties to the family networks and tightly bound churches of the south. Tensions arose due to differences between the teachings of the Canadian evangelical movement and the more conservative beliefs of those who had lived in the south. In some cases, returnees were excommunicated or shunned by their families in the south due to their use of innovations such as automobiles (Quiring, 1997).

This complex migration history is reflected in the significant differences between the Mennonites who have remained in Canada and those who have lived in southern countries. The former typically subscribe to evangelical doctrine, believe that their personal salvation is secure, and expect to enjoy eternal life with God. In comparison, the Mennonites who left for Mexico and other southern countries are not confident that their salvation is assured. Although they hope to spend eternity in heaven, they believe that only God can determine the ultimate fate of human beings (Guenther, 2004). These differences were evident in my research and will be mentioned in the following chapters.

Over time, Mexico's LG Mennonite population expanded substantially; from an original cohort of 6,000 to 7,000, Quiring (1997) estimates that it numbered between 120,000 and 150,000 by 1996. Not surprisingly, land quickly became scarce, requiring the foundation of sister colonies, not all which were situated in arable areas. As increasing numbers of Mennonites became landless, some were forced to seek employment in other sectors of the fast-growing economy, particularly in the Cuauhtémoc area, where they could work in its cheese factories and apple orchards (Quiring, 1997). The Cuauhtémoc Mennonites also began to establish their own businesses. When I visited the region in 2010, I saw how far the group had come. The four-lane highway that runs through part of the main community is dotted with various Mennonite-owned businesses, including furniture-making enterprises, welding and mechanic shops, and recreational facilities such as a skating rink and a number of restaurants.

In his most recent book, *Village among Nations: "Canadian" Mennonites in a Transnational World, 1916–2006,* respected Mennonite scholar Royden Loewen (2013) presents a detailed discussion of the movement of LG Mennonites from Saskatchewan and Manitoba to Central and South America. He carefully links their movement to the history of Canada, while demonstrating how their transnational lives contributed to their uniqueness as a religious group. He estimates that 250,000 LG Mennonites live in North and South America, of which only about one-third remain in the same location as their immediate forebears. More than 20 percent of the LG Mennonites who relocated to Mexico and Paraguay returned to Canada (Loewen, 2013). Not all the Mennonites who returned to Canada stayed permanently; some go back for visits and maintain connections with their relatives (Loewen, 2013).

Through their experiences in these countries, the LG Mennonite groups developed various subtle and more obvious differences. Their complicated history serves as a backdrop to the case study discussed in this book.

Terminology

The complexity of Mennonite history is compounded by the assortment of names used to describe the group, particularly those applied to the Low German Mennonites. It is important to understand that these terms are "cultural" designators and do not identify particular religious groups; LG Mennonites include a range of religious affiliations.

Those who are called Kanadiers are part of the original Old Colony group that came to Canada from Russia during the 1870s and 1880s (Loewen, 1993; Janzen, 2004).[2] Russlanders are Russian Mennonites who migrated to Canada in the 1920s. Some scholars have suggested that the Kanadiers were poorer and more hesitant about social change than the Russlanders (Janzen, 2007; Quiring, 1997). The Russlanders also placed fewer restrictions on the use of modern technologies and on participation in public education (Smith, 1981).

The Mennonites who left Canada for Mexico toward the end of the First World War became known as Mexican Mennonites. After they returned to Canada, this name persisted, but when it fell out of favour, the group asked to be referred to as Low German-speaking Mennonites. In recent years, however, the shorter version "Low German Mennonites" is often used.

Some texts automatically assume that all LG Mennonites are Old Colony Mennonites (the most conservative group in Chortitza, the oldest colony in Russia; Quiring, 1997). Other writers use "Dietsche speakers" to signify all Mennonites who return to Canada from Latin America, regardless of church affiliation (Fehr Keller, 2006; Gingrich, 2013). Some individuals – including Mennonites who live in Canada – believe that Old Colony and Low German Mennonites are one and the same because the most conservative groups tended to leave Canada and stay in countries such as Mexico; my research revealed that "Low German" is often used as an umbrella term to encompass various Mennonite church groups. Over the years, the proliferation of labels has produced confusion, with the result that it is often unclear whether authors of various reports and publications are referring to the same or different groups.

In this book, I follow the lead of Mennonite Central Committee Canada in using "Low German Mennonite." More specifically, the name refers to individuals who moved to Mexico, Belize, and other Latin American countries such as Bolivia and Paraguay during the 1920s and have their roots in the Old Colony Church (Guenther, 2004).

Population

Determining the number of LG Mennonites in Canada and abroad is difficult.[3] Because they have not conformed to the typical migration patterns of refugees or immigrants, precise statistics are not available.

According to John Janzen, former Low German coordinator for Mennonite Central Committee Canada, there were about 250,000 LG Mennonites worldwide in 2010, of which approximately 80,000 lived in Mexico and 10,000 in Belize (Gingrich & Loewen, 2013). Janzen put the number of Canadian LG Mennonites at about 80,000 to 100,000, of which some 40,000 to 50,000 resided in Ontario, 15,000 in Manitoba, and 12,000 to 15,000 in southern Alberta (Janzen, 2010). As of 2015, Janzen suggested that the worldwide population sat at about 350,000. Unsubstantiated estimates suggest that there are 130,000 LG Mennonites in Mexico, 130,000 in Bolivia, and just over 100,000 in Canada, approximately 55,000 of whom live in Ontario, 30,000 in Manitoba, and 25,000 to 30,000 in Alberta.

Religious Variation

A faith-based community can be defined as "an assembly of people (or congregation) whose beliefs about God combine with a common identity, shared history, regular worship, and common values to effect personal and social transformation" (Anderson, 1990, quoted in Hickman, 2006, p. 94). The LG Mennonite history of migration in pursuit of religious and educational freedom, their emphasis on living by shared values, and their common beliefs illustrate that they are principally a faith-based community rather than a cultural group. Importantly, their principles set them apart from others, a fact that has often fostered misunderstandings between themselves and the wider population. In some cases, it has also resulted in discrimination from non-Mennonites.

Mennonites believe that they should adhere to the Ordnung, a set of unwritten rules and guidelines that dictates behaviour (Plasil, 2009). The Ordnung helps them to retain their separateness from the outside world. As Visser (2009) so aptly notes, every generation of Mennonites must choose whether to accept change and become more modern or to reject it and continue to live in the solitude and suffering that are shared by the group.

If an LG Mennonite community decides to reject change, one thing is certain: its members must contribute to and preserve the ways of the group. Community control over personal freedom is important (Driedger, 2000). Consequently, what is and is not acceptable with regards to clothing, behaviour, and activities is clearly defined (Plasil, 2009). Mennonites have traditionally associated the urban environment with dangers that can negatively influence them (Urry, 2006). Their choice to live in rural areas also facilitates the monitoring of individuals and ensures that they will adhere to group norms (Driedger, 2000).

There are several congregational churches within which LG Mennonites worship, and they vary in beliefs and practices. The most conservative have made a steadfast commitment to minimize change and maintain their traditional ways, whereas their more liberal counterparts willingly adapt their religious values and practices to the society around them. The conservative churches include the Old Colony Mennonite Church, whose official name was the Rheinlander Church (Loewen, 2013), and the Sommerfelder Church. The liberal churches, which are based in evangelism, include the Evangelical Mennonite

Church (formerly the Kleine Gemeinde) and the Evangelical Mennonite Mission Church (Guenther, 2004). If individuals or families change churches, they tend to choose one that is more liberal, often because they view the principles and restrictions of the more conservative church as oppressive (Guenther, 2004). Throughout my research, we asked all respondents about their past and current church membership; in all cases, those who had changed churches opted for a more liberal one. Guenther (2004) also notes that a high percentage of LG Mennonites do not participate in a formal church organization.

In general, Mennonite churches originated as splinter groups, the product of schisms within the Old Colony Church and among other congregations. This process has occurred for well over two hundred years; even in Russia during the early nineteenth century, groups sometimes disagreed, and splits accommodated their differences in opinion (Plasil & Roessingh, 2009). Our fieldwork found that geography was linked with church practices; for instance, the Old Colony churches of Alberta have much in common with Old Colony churches in Mexico and are less liberal than Old Colony churches in Manitoba. We attributed this discrepancy to diversity among the leadership: the Alberta leaders are often born, raised, and educated in Mexico, whereas those in Manitoba are often born, raised, and educated in Canada.

One common feature among congregations is their reliance on the Bible as the only truth, the sole way of identifying and following the will of God. Members of conservative churches depend on the bishop and ministers for Biblical interpretation and guidance (Enns, 2009), and are typically not encouraged to read Scripture for themselves. Sometimes, they are even directed not to read it. To complicate matters, Low German is largely a spoken language; only recently have dictionaries (Rempel, 1984; Zacharias, 2009) and the Bible become available in Plautdietsch. In general, therefore, the *Aeltester* (bishop) and ministers – who are chosen for life – interpret the Bible for their congregations, who are not allowed to question the interpretation. Thus, the church plays an important and ongoing role in people's daily lives, and it determines how they will dress and behave, whether they use modern or electrical technology, and a host of other matters.

The most conservative LG Mennonites share a common view of education: they deem it important only to the extent that it prepares individuals for membership in their community; it is not intended to make them members of the state. Public education is seen as encouraging people to question their religious beliefs and the church system to which they belong. It is also seen as promoting competition and pride – traits that are discouraged. Mennonites believe in the importance of humility and feel that individuals who strive for personal accomplishments set themselves apart from the group, causing disharmony and inter-group problems (Quiring, 1997). Generally speaking, most LG Mennonites who move from Mexico to Canada have the equivalent of a Grade 3 or 4 education.

Old Colony Mennonites, who originally comprised the bulk of the LG Mennonite population, believe that properly adhering to their faith requires them to separate themselves from the rest of the world. This does not mean that they must literally live apart, but that they must respect the boundaries and rules that distinguish them from the non-Mennonites in their vicinity. It is important to note that other LG Mennonite groups, from the conservative (such as the Sommerfelder) to the more liberal (such as the Evangelical Mennonite Church), do not necessarily share this belief.

To achieve physical separation, Old Colony Church leaders work to ensure conformity with the Ordnung. They limit personal behaviour and issue long lists of items that parishioners are forbidden to own. The lists vary by church but can include musical instruments, radios, and vehicles equipped with rubber tires – including cars and tractors. Quiring (1997) points out that using a banned object is assumed to weaken adherence to the principles of the church; it is not necessarily the banned object that is the issue, but the disobedience of the church principles that is the concern. He notes the Mennonite belief that use of some modern devices would lead to corrupting influences; for example, vehicles with rubber tires enable transportation to nearby towns that sell alcohol. Radios connect people to the outside world, with its multitude of temptations. Other scholars agree with this interpretation and explain that if such restrictions were not imposed, the rules could easily be changed and the system that protects LG Mennonites from the world would no longer exist (Plasil, 2009). However, the rules are sometimes modified, depending on time and place: for example, Canadian churches have stopped banning the use of rubber tires, although churches in parts of Mexico continue to do so.

The more extensive the list of restrictions, of course, the greater the number of temptations. Old Colony Church leaders see excommunication as an appropriate punishment for those who fail to resist; transgressors lose their standing in the community, and their excommunication or loss of privileges also serves as a deterrent, encouraging everyone else to conform.[4] The practice of excommunication varies from Mexico and other Latin American countries to Canada, where there is more leniency regarding acceptable behaviour. Church leaders cite the Bible to justify the practice, specifically Matthew 16:19, which states, "I will give you the keys of the kingdom of heaven, whatever you bind on earth will be bound in heaven, and whatever you loose on earth will be loosed in heaven!" Though no longer common, excommunication is primarily meted out to men because in this patriarchal society, wives and children are expected to follow the man's lead (Quiring, 1997). At times, large numbers of simultaneous excommunications have occurred (as many as seventy) but without the desired effect, in part because such a large group may create a new, separate community or migrate to Canada in order to avoid the consequences of excommunication. In 1997, researcher David Quiring detected growing dissatisfaction with church leaders in Mexico, which was so intense that the dissenters considered moving back to Canada rather than conforming to the leadership's directives.

In LG Mennonite communities, what women wear depends on their congregation's interpretation of Scripture. For example, Old

Colony Mennonite women and those in other conservative churches wear a headscarf because doing so will encourage God to answer their prayers. However, women in the Evangelical Mennonite Mission Church are not required to wear the scarf and can also wear makeup and jewellery.

Many LG Mennonites have attended public schools and have even completed post-secondary education to enhance their skills and assist their community. Relocating to a community that is not predominantly Mennonite – and that has many perilous attractions – is not considered a favourable option but is sometimes viewed as necessary to obtain higher education. In 2012, a young Mennonite male from Durango Colony completed medical school, becoming the first Mennonite in Mexico to have achieved such an extensive education.

Contrary to popular belief, not all LG Mennonites are restricted from using modern devices such as cellphones or computers; today, even the most conservative churches permit their use. As Kerry Fast and Rachel Epp Buller (2013) state, Old Colony Mennonites value tradition but this does not mean that they are static. Change has been continual among LG Mennonites, not only in Canada but also in Mexico and other Latin American countries, and it has loosened the expectations of group members. It would be rare to find a Mennonite who does not have a cellphone, and many use computers but may reveal this only to trustworthy acquaintances. In Alberta, I met a female member of a conservative church who used a computer to do her homework for her post-secondary studies. Although her father was a minister, he recognized that her education was important for the community.

Today, technological changes make remaining isolated from mainstream society increasingly difficult to achieve, despite the remote locations in which some LG Mennonites live. The impact of the Internet and social media cannot be overstated; community members express concern that these media provide exposure to ideas or practices that are contrary to LG Mennonite religious beliefs. Such technology also represents a drive toward individualism rather than the communalism that is a main focus of Mennonite life (Driedger, 2000).

Throughout their history, LG Mennonites have migrated in hopes of escaping religious persecution. Their continual movement, desire for separateness, low level of education, and reliance on ministerial assistance have generated misconceptions regarding their beliefs and practices. Such misunderstandings can affect their interactions with health care and social service providers, among others. An understanding of the history, beliefs, and practices of the LG Mennonite community will help health provides who wish to work with this unique group.

2

HEALTH AND ILLNESS

My first study with Low German Mennonites took place in southern Alberta in 2000 (Hall & Kulig, 2004; Hall et al., 2005; Kulig et al., 2002; Kulig & Hall, 2004). Its purpose was to compile information about this group's beliefs and practices surrounding health and illness. The eighty-six participants (forty-one males and forty-five females) were interviewed in their homes by trained research assistants (RAs). The perspectives presented here are primarily from this sample; however, because we asked participants in our other studies about their views on health, some of their responses are also included here. Unless otherwise stated, the focus is on what LG Mennonites in Canada believe and experience.

Interviewee responses varied according to church affiliation and length of residency in Canada. Not unexpectedly, the most conservative individuals who had been in Canada for the shortest time had the greatest difficulty in expressing their ideas. When they did, we learned that they were more likely than those from more established communities to have held on to their traditional views. In contrast, those who had lived in Canada for longer (generally more than five years) were more comfortable in conversing with us. They were affiliated with liberal churches, and their beliefs had begun to adapt to those of mainstream Canadians.

Regardless of their backgrounds, however, all shared certain attitudes about health. For example, they understood that there were inherent differences between men's and women's health. Although human anatomy and physiology were not taught in many of their private schools and were not part of their curriculum, they recognized that because women bore children, they had certain health problems that did not affect men. They rarely saw dental health as an important part of overall health. In sharing their understanding of health and illness, suffering, and the treatment of illness, they painted a vivid picture of their beliefs and world view.

Defining Health and Illness

How our interviewees defined health varied from one location to another. They described being healthy as having energy and strength, and being pain-free. People who enjoyed good health were motivated, independent, and able to work. According to one participant, being healthy meant not being greedy. Another said that "illness is the absence or failure to cultivate the gift [of life that] God has given."

In contrast, Kerstin Reinschmidt (2001) found that community members in Mexico did not focus overtly on health; instead, they saw it in terms of the ability to work. Illness was associated with being unable to work, a situation that was uncommon and undesirable, as the community's rural lifestyle depended upon the capacity of women and men to carry on their duties both within and outside the home. The interviewees in Reinschmidt's study described three states of health: a "healthy" individual was capable of working; a "sickly" person could be a hypochondriac or someone whose health fluctuated and thus could not always work hard; and a "sick" person was unwell and possibly unable to work. The women also believed that continuing to work would help them get through a period of sickness; illness interfered with their everyday life, so they automatically suppressed their symptoms, ignoring them and continuing to work. This behaviour also helped them to preserve their good moral standing in the community.

In the late 1990s, Elizabeth Burrill (1998) researched Mennonite families who came from Mexico but were living in southwestern Ontario. She focused on health perceptions, family health work, and health-promoting lifestyle practices. In her study, thirty-six LG Mennonite mothers completed a structured interview, which included the Health Options Scale (a measure of how families work together to promote their health) and the Health-Promoting Lifestyle Profile II (a questionnaire that measures behaviours related to health). Six mothers from the original sample participated in a second semi-structured interview regarding their health and health-promotion strategies. Burrill found that they identified three categories of health: physical, mental, and spiritual. This was similar to our findings, discussed below.

Values Related to Health

Three values regarding health emerged from our interviews as being especially significant to LG Mennonites: cleanliness, nutrition, and psychological health.

Participants often commented on the importance of good hygiene for the body and the home. The women devoted most of their time to domestic chores, caring for their homes, themselves, and their children. Maintaining standards of cleanliness in houses that lack running water, as can be the case in Mexico and other southern locales, is no small task, particularly when large families are involved. In one instance, we became disturbed about over-cleanliness when we learned that women in Belize were washing their walls with diluted dichlorodiphenyltrichloroethane (DDT) to reduce the incidence of insects; although studies into the negative effects of DDT on human health, including on fetuses, are inconsistent, there is enough evidence to cause concern about exposure (Kezios et al., 2013). This practice points to the need to conduct thorough health histories with Mennonite women who move to Canada.

LG Mennonite women place a high priority on feeding their families good and nutritious food. They are well known for their baking but also make sausages and cheese, and are accustomed to raising chickens and dairy cattle. In Mexico, LG Mennonites have added tortillas to their diets, which are a mainstay for those who relocate to Canada. Mennonite stores in Canada sell tinned foods from Mexico and fresh items such as chili peppers that have become commonplace in meal preparation.

LG Mennonites value psychological health in everyday life. Throughout our studies, interviewees commented on the importance of reducing stress and being happy, and on the crucial benefits of maintaining a positive attitude when facing health challenges and for health in general. They associated psychological health with spiritual health, a connection that necessitated a relationship with God. How personal this relationship should be depended upon church affiliation, with more liberal members fostering a closer, more intimate relationship than those in conservative churches.

Although they value clean living, LG Mennonites are not immune from engaging in unhealthy practices. Some adults smoke, a habit that has become more common among youth – girls as well as boys. Substance abuse, including alcoholism, has become a serious concern because it runs counter to the group's religious principles. LG Mennonites who move to Canada have changed their diets, sometimes in unwholesome ways, due to financial constraints or failure to understand nutritional requirements. This is especially evident among children and young families; teachers have noted that, like children from mainstream society, LG Mennonite children may bring inappropriate lunches to school, citing hot dogs and Kool-Aid as examples. Behaviours ranging from neglect to alcohol abuse to domestic violence have caused great stress in some homes, despite the emphasis among all Mennonites on peace (Penner, 1999).

Understanding Illness

When we asked participants to identify overarching categories for individual health problems, they often found it difficult to do so. However, they did list problems that they or others in their community had experienced, such as arthritis, cancer, heart disease, and the baby blues. When our RAs spoke with them about inherited diseases, their replies showed that they were aware of the links between diseases and family members. However, they used the phrase "through the blood" rather than terms such as "genetically transmitted." Our thematic analysis revealed three categories of illness: physical, mental, and spiritual. We spoke with the Mennonite RAs and the advisory team, who confirmed that these categories fit with the data that had been generated in the interviews and discussions with participants.

Physical Illness

One interviewee referred to physical illness as "being from the flesh and bone." Women, men, and children all experienced it. When we asked participants to name physical illnesses, they listed arthritis, diabetes, broken bones, high blood pressure, cancer, and acute conditions such as strep throat. They frequently mentioned *Kopp Krankheit*, referring to children whose heads were disproportionately large compared to their bodies – probably the result of malnutrition.

Some respondents believed that health problems crossed between categories and that physical illnesses could also be psychologically or spiritually based. For instance, heart problems could be seen as a sign of troubles caused by Satan, a "troubled heart," or the result of a bad relationship.

Through her interviews and participant observation in Mexico, Reinschmidt (2001) assembled a list of diseases that LG Mennonites experienced and noted. For the most part, they were common to virtually all human populations – including cancer, heart disease, and arthritis. However, unlike in mainstream society, many were connected to Mexico's harsh climate and to agricultural work. For example, burns were common, associated with washing clothes by hand, and farm accidents were frequent among the men.

Mental Illness

Respondents recognized that women, men, and children could suffer from mental illness, and they felt that someone who was sad or worried would be prone to it. These emotions could arise from problems in the home, such as alcohol issues or financial difficulties. "Having nerves" *(narvenkrankheit)* and being depressed were also frequently mentioned. Here, a link was made between the person's heart and mental illness: if one's heart did not belong to God, it could belong to Satan, and the individual would experience a heavy heart, have nerves, or become mentally ill. A firm faith in God was crucial to mental health. Furthermore, someone who was not mentally well and continued to worry excessively could turn to angry and abusive behaviours, exacerbating an already difficult situation.

Our initial findings on this topic and the way in which the theme of mental illness recurred in two subsequent studies (on women's sexuality and death and dying), led us to undertake a stand-alone study on mental health and illness. The findings of that study are discussed in Chapter 5.

Spiritual Illness

It is not uncommon for researchers to differentiate between physical and mental illness, but our study was unique in its need to establish spiritual illness as a third formal category. Interviewees believed that it was caused by Satan or by nerve problems. Drifting away from God gave Satan the opportunity to fill a person's heart, which could result in inappropriate behaviours such as substance abuse. Interviewees recognized that such abuse would lead to physical problems, as well as having negative impacts on emotional and psychological health – not only on themselves but on others. For example, in homes where the husband had a substance abuse problem, money was allocated to alcohol rather than groceries, and the wife and children might be subject to violence. Clergymen sometimes intervened by providing groceries and by talking with the husband about his spiritual failings. They also offered to pray with him and gave additional counselling if he showed a willingness to change. Our interviewees understood that an individual could be helped only if he or she were willing to make changes and be helped. Their feeling that prayer was necessary for individuals with substance abuse problems illustrated their belief in the significance of spiritual healing.

Perceptions of Suffering

Suffering was a common theme in all my research with LG Mennonites (Kulig & Fan, 2011), and consideration of this topic is fundamental to understanding them. Their attitudes toward suffering permeate all aspects of their beliefs in relation to health and illness, including the three areas we studied: women's health, death and dying, and mental health. The care strategies and activities of LG Mennonites were intended to reduce their own suffering and that of others.

LG Mennonites see suffering as a natural part of life. In his Bolivia research, Lorenzo Cañás Bottos (2008) notes that they conceive of life in terms of two alternative paths. The first entails embracing suffering as a way of imitating Christ and remaining separate from the world. This path is difficult because those who follow it must attend church, heed the voice of God, and pray for mercy. The second path involves yielding to the temptations of Satan, including physical desires. Its ultimate end is damnation. Similarly, Reinschmidt (2001) describes suffering as having religious and moral significance in the daily lives of Mexican-based LG Mennonites.

Our respondents' understanding of suffering – dealing with difficult times or events in their lives – depended on the church to which they belonged. The most conservative were certain that suffering was sent by God. One man said, "It's a test. Because we don't listen to God." For this man and others like him, suffering could teach a lesson, and the proper response to it could bring one closer to God. For example, the birth of a child with disabilities gave its family the opportunity to care for it in a manner that exemplified their acceptance of the situation. When God allowed LG Mennonites to experience events that caused suffering, they could use it to develop their relationship with him. This was sometimes referred to as "having a cross to bear," and the examples ranged from the mothers of disabled children to individuals with substance abuse problems. In these instances, the Mennonites felt that God suffered along with his people; he did not allow them to suffer alone. One participant said, "God allows us to suffer so that people's faith can be strengthened, and that seems to be part of the reason why we suffer on earth." Another stated, "Yes, and that's what we're here for, to suffer with our Lord, and when I've suffered enough, God will take me home." Another commented, "I sometimes have to be sick to reflect on God and to pray more." Our interviewees saw illness as a form of suffering that tested their faith and they felt that choosing to act outside the principles of the church could lead to suffering. Reflecting on the connections between illness and lifestyle choices, and either accepting the illness or changing one's behaviour, could lead to a closer relationship with God, a worthy goal for any LG Mennonite.

According to one participant, "It was not God's original plan for us to suffer, but now it is part of our life because of sin entering the world in the Garden of Eden." Interviewees insisted that God did not actually inflict suffering; instead, everyone experienced issues that could produce it. One said,

> I don't think it is always God's will that we suffer. But sometimes suffering does the people good, because that way they often get to see their sinful life and they change their life around. Sometimes lengthy illnesses are a kind of suffering, but if death is a kind of suffering, I am not so sure about it, because we don't know.

Although participants saw God as benevolent, they believed that human sinfulness could prompt him to mete out punishment. Because humans were sinful, they could and did make choices that deviated from their religious principles. In these instances, suffering was the result of their decisions and was not preordained by God. In the

Bible, Hebrews 12:11 states, "Now, discipline always seems painful rather than pleasant at the time, but later it yields the peaceful fruit of righteousness to those who have been trained by it." By suffering, people could draw on their strength to endure and acknowledge God's positive role in their lives. Suffering was also an opportunity to accept and deal with their lives, including addressing their poor choices. Through this reflection, they could reform their behaviour while also growing closer to God.

A Bolivian Mennonite whom we interviewed said, "It is not God's will if we suffer, and it certainly isn't God's will that we worry a lot." Another said that suffering was not given by God – it was the result of bad decisions that people made. Still another explained that when individuals stray from God, the Devil attracts them and sways them to make inappropriate choices, such as becoming alcoholics. A minister stated, "God did not want us to suffer, but sin brought it upon us." The participants often expanded upon this idea by talking about alcoholism. One mentioned an alcoholic who caused the death of his family members while driving drunk. His decision to drink was seen as a sinful behaviour and as the direct cause of the deaths. Interviewees believed that living one's life "improperly" led to physical or spiritual suffering for oneself and others. Making inappropriate choices, such as consuming alcohol, rather than turning to God for help would ultimately leave a person with a heavy heart and vulnerable to the temptations of Satan. Women and children would also suffer if the father were unable to work and provide for them or if he were physically or emotionally abusive. Their suffering enabled them to draw on their strength in dealing with their circumstances. Hopefully, the father would acknowledge the sinfulness of his behaviour and make the necessary changes.

In our study of death and dying, participants discussed both the physical and the spiritual aspects of suffering, including pain, loss of mobility, and the inability to converse with others. Medications such as painkillers were accepted treatments but were not seen as the only remedy for physical suffering: prayer could also reduce pain. Some respondents interpreted pain as flagging a "spiritually unresolved problem." In such instances, the minister would be crucial in helping individuals to deal with their spiritual issue, thereby relieving the pain.

Even when suffering was associated with dying, interviewees emphasized that it was "spiritual suffering," a necessary part of preparing to meet death. In this context, it was not seen as negative, because it helped individuals ready themselves for death and for eternal life: the desired outcome. In fact, it was beneficial, enabling dying individuals to restore and deepen their relationship with God and to receive forgiveness for their sins. If they sincerely atoned for their sins and achieved salvation, death would release them from physical pain and spiritual suffering.

Health Treatments

Studies show that, much like members of wider society, LG Mennonites seek and combine various remedies for illness, ranging from traditional home cures, to care from bone-setters, to treatment by physicians and other providers in the mainstream system (Reinschmidt, 2001; Burrill, 1998; Kulig & Hall, 2004).

Reinschmidt (2001) found that LG Mennonites in Mexico followed a routine in dealing with disease and injuries. First, they tried their own home remedies, such as herbs and teas. If these failed to work, they sought assistance from a community member, such as a bone-setter (whom community members sometimes referred to as a chiropractor). During pregnancy, they consulted the local Mennonite midwives. If these treatments proved ineffective, they resorted to mainstream practitioners, including Mexican physicians or the sole Mennonite doctor who was available at that time. Seeing a Mexican physician was complicated, not only because the clinic lay some distance away but also due to the need for translation – which, for women, was often provided by the husband and may or may not have been accurate in conveying either symptoms to the physician or treatment to the patient. LG Mennonites simultaneously used both their own home remedies and prescriptions or other treatments provided by licensed health care practitioners. My fieldwork in Mexico uncovered a similar pattern: LG Mennonites often mixed treatments – not unlike other groups, including mainstream Canadians who combine prescription drugs with vitamins, herbs, and other natural products.

In her studies in southern Ontario, Elizabeth Burrill (1998) found that LG Mennonite families relied on their own knowledge and skills in dealing with signs and symptoms when they first appeared, and sought out the expert opinion of physicians if the illness were not resolved. There was little emphasis on setting goals to meet health priorities. The women whom Burrill interviewed stated that spiritual growth was met through church and community involvement and by sustaining healthy interpersonal relationships, an important component of health.

Our studies in Canada indicated that health treatments could be divided into physical and spiritual categories, much like health conditions themselves. A number of alternative treatments were used on their own or in combination with prescription drugs. However, unlike mainstream Canadians, LG Mennonites take a transnational approach to care: they access certain Mexican products that are not readily available in Canada. They may purchase these when they visit family in Mexico, or friends and relatives may bring them back to Canada. A growing number of Canadian stores now offer these products, reducing the necessity of bringing them from Mexico.

Physical treatments for individuals of all ages included pills or creams and salves, many of whose ingredients were unknown to us. For example, Doctor Thomas Electric liniment and ZMO Oil were both suggested for arthritic pain, and Metamizol Sodico or inhaling vapours were recommended for toothache. Bee salve was also used for arthritic pain. There were a number cold remedies, including rubbing Wonder Oil and China Oil (a mint product that smelled like ammonia) on ears and throats. Dandelion roots could also be helpful in treating a cold. Diarrhea and vomiting could be relieved by such products as Hieng Fong (mint drops, a multipurpose item that was also useful for bee stings and toothache). Cuts could be treated with pine oil, and gun grease could relieve eczema. Chamomile was frequently mentioned as useful for stomach cramps and discomfort.

Interviewees talked about mixing Canadian and Mexican treatments, including prescription antibiotics and over-the-counter medicines. In Mexico and Belize, they could purchase a wide array of prescription drugs over the counter, although at least in Mexico this practice is now changing; antibiotics, hormone shots, and painkillers were easily obtainable in the city or local pharmacias. The Mennonite-run pharmacias that I observed in Mexico and Belize sold a range of drugs over the counter – including antibiotics and analgesics – even though the manager had little pharmaceutical education; Reinschmidt (2001) made a similar observation. Pharmacias also sold first aid essentials such as bandages, and they stocked mobility aids, such as canes and crutches.

Interviewees understood that mixing Canadian and Mexican medications might not be wise, and some admitted that physicians had discouraged it. Some had developed a complicated procedure for using both kinds of treatment. One woman used a Canadian prescription until it ran out and then switched to a Mexican treatment, or vice versa. This whole topic proved very complex. Some perceived that Mexican oral medications should not be taken but that external salves and creams would be safe. Some felt that mixing Mexican and Canadian medicines was dangerous, even if their use were staggered. This variety of conflicting information illustrates the necessity for health care professionals to ask LG Mennonites whether they are mixing medicines.

Among LG Mennonite families who arrive in Canada from places such as Mexico and Belize, assumptions regarding care often differ from those of the Canadian-born. For example, they commonly expect that visiting a doctor will involve being given medication of some kind. Because they can so easily purchase drugs in the south, including antibiotics, which are available over the counter, and because they lack a scientific understanding of disease, they are not always satisfied with the care they receive at Canadian health clinics.

The participants also employed folk remedies. Tonsillitis could be cured by pulling a specific hair on the afflicted person's head, which would rip away the nerve that had caused the problem; some who had experienced this treatment said that they could hear the nerve tear. Feverish children were given scalded milk. Burns were treated with cloths soaked in varnish to remove the dead skin, after which cottage cheese drippings were placed on the burned area. Some interviewees soaked avocado pits in oil and made a liniment for arthritis pain. Others soaked cloths in sour cream and placed them on arthritic joints to combat pain. Several believed that reducing the intake of yeast products relieved arthritis, a difficult remedy to apply given the community's large consumption of homemade breads.

Participants told us that a physician in Mexico provided injections that helped stop alcoholism. However, the injection was effective for only five years, and one interviewee mentioned a friend who had returned to drinking once the five years ended. Another unusual treatment applied to Kopp Krankheit. The children who suffered from this condition were given corn tortillas that had been soaked in calcium and lime juice, which suggests an underlying belief that the disorder was related to nutritional deficiency.

In addition to using their own alternative treatments, interviewees could consult alternative health providers in their adopted Canadian communities. Some of these individuals developed their skills in Mexico or Belize and continued to practise after moving to Canada. One of these providers, who specialized in women's health, was called a "lady doctor," although she had no formal training.[1]

In Mexico, LG Mennonite health providers managed ailments among the community and attempted to restore sick and injured individuals to health. In Durango Colony, which had several of these practitioners, I observed a bone-setter as she conducted a diagnosis and treatment session for a patient with knee pain. She had been an active healer for decades, and she saw her patients in a small room at her home. Using her hands, she palpated the patient's knee to assess the pain and reach a diagnosis. Her treatment primarily involved vitamins and minerals. Practitioners such as this bone-setter are paid a small amount of money for their skill. I also met a woman who had taken various short courses on topics such as physiotherapy and dispensing drugs. She sold over-the-counter medication to anyone who requested it, and her clinic included physiotherapy equipment to help individuals in their rehabilitation.

Caregiving Roles

In general, the daily lives of LG Mennonites are expected to be spiritually sound and morally upright, in obedience to the word of God as expressed in the Bible and directed through the church. The caregiving that occurs in families exemplifies this manner of living and helps bolster community solidarity. The family is primarily responsible for raising the children and for caring for aging parents. When children or youth become ill or are injured, parents must seek care and provide whatever measures are possible to address the problem. The mother is the principal caregiver. In Mexico and other southern countries, including Belize, caregivers obtain medications and other treatments from pharmacias and LG Mennonite health providers.

In Canada, the mother often experiences challenges in accessing care. For instance, her English will commonly be limited, so explaining symptoms and answering questions will be difficult. Simply getting to the clinic or hospital can be a problem, as she will rely on her husband for transportation, but his work schedule may conflict with clinic hours.

In southern Alberta, LG Mennonite liaison workers have proved an asset in community health-promotion programs. They drive mothers and their children to clinics and hospitals, and they act as translators. They can also supply crucial explanations to the family about the illness or condition that a health professional has diagnosed and will then do a follow-up to determine that the necessary care is being provided.

In speaking with these liaison workers over the years, I have learned that follow-up home visits often reveal other family issues. The most challenging has been the discovery of children with undiagnosed genetic disorders. In such cases, the liaison worker arranges a number of appointments, including transportation to genetic clinics in larger cities and extensive visits with the family to assist them in caring for the child. Liaison workers may also detect symptoms that need further exploration, such as symptoms of undiagnosed type 1 diabetes in young children. Such a diagnosis requires home visits to teach the family about the dietary needs of the child and the use of injectable insulin and other medications.

In Mexico, where houses are often too small to accommodate extended families, care homes for the aged (Altenheim) have been established in which each person lives in a private room and eats in a shared dining room. The decision to create these facilities was made at the community level (Quiring, 1997). On the weekend, the dining room is open to members of the wider community, who are welcome to eat there; profits from the sale of their meals are used to maintain the facility. These homes also provide employment for local women, who cook, clean, and supply personal care.

A similar approach to caring for the elderly is evolving in Canadian Mennonite communities. In Winkler, Manitoba, for example, a care facility named Salem Home is based on principles of the Mennonite churches. Salem Home accepts non-Mennonites, but Mennonite ministers and church members in good standing sit on its board, helping to direct the care and services that it provides. The issue of elder care has also arisen among LG Mennonite groups in southern Alberta, some of whom feel that a care facility should be built to house elderly LG Mennonites. Conversely, some LG Mennonite families in this area prefer to care for their aged parents at home.

LG Mennonites in Mexico also founded care facilities for individuals with developmental or mental health disabilities. I visited two such facilities – one in the Cuauhtémoc area and one at Durango

Colony, in 2010 and 2012, respectively. Both housed residents whose conditions ranged from schizophrenia, to fetal alcohol spectrum disorder, to Down's syndrome. They had private rooms. A single person or a couple ran the facility, and young women helped with the everyday chores such as cooking and cleaning. The residents were expected to participate in various activities or carry out certain tasks, depending upon their ability. The Cuauhtémoc facility had a wood shop in which the men made furniture that was sold to the public. Young female residents made rugs and other items that were also sold, and the profits from all these sales helped to manage the facility.

When a person of any age requires care at home, family members – mostly the females – attend to his or her physical needs. This practice continues when the individual is admitted to hospital or a facility. LG Mennonites typically refrain from complaining about the care that health professionals supply (Fan, 2011). Thus, practitioners and managers who want feedback from LG Mennonites must broach the subject with family members, while also ensuring that they understand why care is being provided in the manner that it is.

The understandings of health and illness among LG Mennonites are based in shared values and include the interdependence of physical, mental, and spiritual categories. Health treatments need to match these perspectives but are also contingent upon the availability of resources, including traditional and professional providers. Caregiving is an important role for women, but engaging in it also enables LG Mennonites to honour the principle of aiding others while contributing to community well-being.

3

WOMEN'S HEALTH

Among Low German Mennonites, beliefs and practices related to the health of women vary from one church to another and from one geographic area to another. A main reason for this is that ministers do not necessarily agree in their interpretation of the Bible, which ultimately determines the health behaviours of their congregational members. The issue is further complicated because individual Mennonites may opt to disregard the guidance of the church and make their own choices, with or without the knowledge of their minister. In the case of women, the church can provide varying degrees of support, leading to a range of health consequences for them and their families.

As part of my research, we interviewed thirty-eight women about their beliefs and knowledge related to sexuality, including sexual and reproductive health and their needs for health promotion about this topic (Kulig et al., 2006; Kulig et al., 2008; Kulig et al., 2009). We also gleaned information from LG Mennonite women during our other studies in the community; the findings presented here come from all of them.

Because women's health could be such a sensitive topic, we took great care to make interviewees feel comfortable and safe in talking to me and the research assistants. Many told us that the interview was their first opportunity to discuss their feelings about the subject or how their bodies worked. They found the interviews enlightening, said that they had learned about their bodies, and wanted to know more.

The women ranged in age from early twenties to eighties, and their opinions varied according to their ages. Collectively, their children had been born in several countries (Mexico, Belize, Bolivia, and Canada) from the 1940s to the early 2000s; in other words, they had given birth and raised children over a wide range of time periods and in many social contexts. Some had been born in Mexico, Belize, or Bolivia and had moved to a Canadian province, some had lived in the United States, and some had lived only in Mexico. Their perspectives reflected a range of beliefs and practices and may have changed over the course of their lives. The women represented a variety of Mennonite church memberships, and a number of them had changed churches at some point in their lives.

Women's Roles in Family and Community Life

Until recently, little information had been published about LG Mennonite women. The historical documents that do exist indicate that they are "either dependent on men or helpless in their absence" (Loewen, 2001, p. 53). In general, LG Mennonites see women as the weaker sex: Loewen concluded that a woman's role was to silently support her husband and bear many children, while simultaneously focusing on running the house. In an influential article titled "Women in Canadian Mennonite History: Uncovering the 'Underside,'" Mennonite historian Marlene Epp (1987) highlighted the lack of emphasis on the importance of Mennonite women *as women* in the historical development of this group; instead, they have traditionally been discussed in terms of their influence on men. Their hesitancy, quietness, and modesty ensure that their opinions and ideas are not openly discussed. When a woman marries, she takes not only her husband's last name but also his first, which reinforces her lack of a separate identity: when Miss Anna Friesen becomes Mrs. John Toews, the change not only identifies the man to whom she is married but also erases her own status as an individual.

Autobiographies and written descriptions of the lives of Mennonite women confirm the importance and nature of their roles in their households and communities. A common theme of these accounts is the hard work required of both women and men. Living in Mexico or Belize or migrating across Canada to isolated locales such as La Crete, Alberta, meant that they enjoyed few conveniences, and the price of economic success for families and communities was constant labour by everyone.

One LG Mennonite woman, Helena Wiebe Krahn (2012), wrote a personal account of such a life. Born in Durango in 1932, Wiebe Krahn eventually married and moved several times between Mexico and Ontario. To succeed in her marriage and to be part of her community, she took the approach of simply accepting negative events, such as house fires, loss of family members, employment challenges, and dissension in the church. When she wrote her memoirs, she was in her seventies, widowed, and residing with adult children in a Mennonite community in Tasmania.

For Mennonites, motherhood is a central institution through which beliefs and practices are learned and passed down to subsequent generations (Fast & Epp Buller, 2013). In general, women are defined by family life and by their roles as wives and mothers; these roles are interwoven with those of other family members and ultimately with the community as a whole, which in turn shapes family structures and the roles of others. Furthermore, as mothers, women are expected to abide by the norms of their religious doctrines and communities. They are therefore central to the transmission and conveyance of Mennonite identity (Fast & Epp Buller, 2013).

Previous Studies

Understanding Mennonite perspectives regarding sexuality and women's health was an important aspect of the research that shaped this book. Publications that deal specifically with LG Mennonite views on this topic are very scarce. Much of the literature is dated and may no longer be applicable.

Theologian Brenda Hurst (2003) examined Mennonite attitudes regarding sexuality from 1890 to 1930 by reviewing and assessing periodicals, books, records, and sermons from Mennonite Church conferences. Although she did not focus specifically on LG Mennonites, her study shows parallels between their beliefs and those of the Mennonites who formed the Mennonite Church in the United States. Hurst concluded that Mennonites held five basic beliefs related to gender and sexuality: men have authority over women; the sexes have distinct roles due to their differing capabilities; human spiritual nature is more important than physical or sexual nature; reason must govern passion, including sexual desire; and one's duty to God, rather than a desire for pleasure, should motivate sexual behaviour. These beliefs were reinforced by particular acts or expectations regarding behaviour. For instance, after baptism – which occurs during young adulthood – Mennonite women of conservative churches must wear a headscarf at all times; it is commonly thought that God will not hear their prayers unless the scarf is worn. Hurst (2003, p. 101) found that the home was seen as a "paradise in a sinful world," a place where husband and wife could comfort one another as they dealt with the burdens of their independent but interrelated worlds. Sex was to occur only in marriage, and it was believed that the mind could control sexual desire. Church leaders in the 1920s and 1930s taught that women had sexual power over men; importantly, they were responsible for ensuring that men did not become attracted to them. Marriage relieved the loneliness of a man's life, and it was not considered completely happy until it produced children. During this era, women, including mothers, daughters, and female friends, shared little information about female sexuality with each other (Hurst, 2003).

In 1979, George Brenneman published a literature review that examined Mennonite perspectives on abortion. According to him, they believed that God would decide when a pregnancy threatened a woman's life and would terminate it by causing a miscarriage. Opting for an abortion had both an individual and a societal impact, as it deprived the community of a future parishioner (Brenneman, 1979). It is unclear whether present-day LG Mennonites subscribe to these beliefs.

Over thirty years ago, historian Marlene Epp (1987) identified the need for a more comprehensive understanding of historical and current Mennonite views on sexuality – and for more extensive research with Mennonite women, taking into account their roles and influence in the community. Since then, progress has been made on this front. One challenge facing researchers is the range of Mennonite groups and the inappropriateness of making generalizations about them. Until sufficient research is conducted among the full range of Mennonite women, we will not fully understand them.

As Epp (1987) notes, few research studies regarding Mennonite women were conducted during the 1980s, and as I have found, even fewer focus on *Low German* Mennonite women. Studies that attempted to do so sometimes achieved limited success in collecting data. A case in point is a study on family size in Cuauhtémoc's Manitoba Colony (Felt, Ridley, Allen, & Redekop, 1990). Although it supported anecdotal evidence that LG Mennonites have high fertility rates, its results are questionable from a scientific viewpoint due to the low response of the group itself. Community members did not trust the researchers and thus refused to participate in the study.

One exception is Kerstin Reinschmidt's study of LG Mennonite women, including their roles in health and illness, conducted in the Cuauhtémoc area during the 1990s (Reinschmidt, 2001). During her extensive fieldwork (a total of thirteen months) in the Manitoba Colony, she observed LG Mennonite women from two congregations – the conservative Old Colony and the more liberal General Conference. Her interview sample consisted of sixteen General Conference women who represented eleven families and fifteen households; fourteen Old Colony women from two families and eleven households; and twelve health care practitioners, including a Mennonite family physician, seven Mennonite nurses, a female Mennonite healer, and three Mexican doctors.

During her interviews, Reinschmidt became acquainted with many members of the community. She found that women's health issues, such as pregnancy and childbirth, were not openly discussed when unmarried women were present, although married women discussed such topics among themselves. Reinschmidt also learned that women were encouraged to have numerous children. They viewed health in two ways: It was an individual and physical attribute that could be measured by a person's ability to work; in this regard, illnesses could be countered with home remedies and formal medical treatment as necessary. Health was also seen as a moral and spiritual experience that was achieved by living every day in a way that exemplified religious values and beliefs (Reinschmidt, 2001, p. 347). Women were responsible for health care and were charged with ensuring that their families remained healthy, a fact that added to their workload. Because Mennonites value cleanliness and good nutrition, women were expected to maintain spotless homes and to cook healthy food. Preventing farm accidents was also a priority, because the community isolation and lack of resources made it difficult for women to treat life-threatening injuries.

My research showed that most of Reinschmidt's findings remain true today, regardless of whether an LG Mennonite woman lives in Canada, Belize, or Mexico. Women commonly supported each other during times of illness or after childbirth by paying visits to offer advice, provide meals, or assist with chores such as the laundry. Praying for each other was another common support mechanism. Clearly, however, more information is needed about LG Mennonite women to provide appropriate care.

Women's Access to Health Care

Generally speaking, LG Mennonite women who live in Mexico and Belize can use the services of professional health providers (for example, through Christian charity organizations), as well as those of self-taught practitioners who belong to their community. Some women have access to traditional birth attendants, lady doctors, or bone-setters in their villages. These individuals usually treat patients in their homes. They have no formal medical training and are often drawn to service after seeing a relative care for others. They may learn from the relative but are often self-taught. Some practitioners told me that they had benefitted from reading materials on anatomy and physiology.

In some LG Mennonite villages in Mexico and Belize, health services are offered through established clinics by an individual who has basic training in fields such as physiotherapy. The clinic may also sell an assortment of over-the-counter medications. In some parts of Mexico, for instance, the Mennonite Central Committee (MCC) provides a variety of services through volunteer workers from Canada or the United States. These workers may have a nursing background and may thus also provide assistance such as mental health counselling.

LG Mennonite women are also entitled to use their country's mainstream system to see a physician, pharmacist, physiotherapist, or other professional. Whether they can actually access these services depends on the availability of transportation, an ongoing issue for some families due to distance, lack of vehicles, and whether or not a woman is allowed to drive.

In Canada, not every geographic area has a Mennonite health provider such as a lady doctor or a bone-setter, who are more numerous in Latin America. However, LG Mennonite women in Canada have access to a variety of professional health providers at no cost or low cost, due to subsidies for those with low income, through the mainstream system. Here too, transportation and the language barrier remain issues. This reinforces the importance of the Mennonite liaison worker.

Caring for Others

LG Mennonite women see caring for others as a moral duty that is embedded in their commitment to mutual love in their community.

In addition to their day-to-day domestic chores, the women to whom I spoke were responsible for meeting the needs of people in their households, such as husbands, children, parents, grandparents, while also contributing to the care of others in the community.

Throughout my interviews and fieldwork, I found that the lives of LG Mennonite women – particularly those who had lived in Mexico, Belize, Bolivia, Paraguay, and other Latin American countries – were characterized by hard work. When Mennonites first moved to these countries, they needed to create homes and establish themselves in the farming industry. They had little access to health care practitioners or facilities; when health problems arose, the women employed home treatments and relied on prayer.

They had few conveniences. Their everyday chores included baking, cooking, making soap, and doing laundry by hand. The fact that they gave birth every year or two increased their domestic labour. In some families, the husband supported his wife by helping with childcare or housework, but these were exceptions. Some female interviewees said that they had raised their sons to be more helpful around the home and more intimately involved in childcare than their husbands had been, to reduce the workload of future daughters-in-law.

I heard many examples of how LG Mennonite women cared for others as they grew up in Mexico or Belize and after coming to Canada. They provided assistance, such as babysitting or delivering meals, to families dealing with illness or the birth of a baby. They took turns helping out, to ensure that assistance could be sustained for as long as the family needed it.

Caring for Oneself

Our female interviewees devoted most of their energy to caring for others. The little time left for self-care concentrated on sexuality and their health in a general sense. As noted in the literature and confirmed in our interviews, there is virtual silence regarding female sexuality; candid conversations are limited to close confidantes or trusted outsiders.

Among LG Mennonites, an underlying theme related to women's health, particularly sexuality, is the importance of maintaining family honour and respect for the family within the community, which includes their church membership. This honour is defined by Scripture, which describes suitable female behaviour. For example, 1 Timothy 2:11 states, "Let a woman learn in silence with full submission," a verse that is often interpreted to mean that a woman must acquiesce to her father and, when married, to her husband. Furthermore, 2 Thessalonians 2:15 decrees, "So then, brothers and sisters, stand firm and hold fast to the traditions that you were taught by us, either by word of mouth or by our letter." This is taken to mean that change and learning new ideas are not always appropriate. LG Mennonites are encouraged to follow the teachings of their ministers and are thus not exposed to new knowledge, which might prompt them to question behavioural norms and possibly disobey them.

For example, some participants believed that women who learned about sexual intercourse before they married could choose to engage in pre-marital sex, which would degrade family honour. They believed that both women and men could control their sexual desire but that women held sexual power over men. Perhaps contradictorily, they also thought that a woman who refused to have sex with her husband was committing a sin by denying him his rights.

Given the interrelationships among sexuality, family honour, and faith-based expectations regarding behaviour, it is not surprising that knowledge about sexuality and women's health varied. However, we also found that younger LG Mennonite women generally had a better understanding of topics such as family planning and pregnancy than did older women. This pattern mirrors that of other groups, including mainstream Canadians, where youth have the advantage of higher education and more exposure to information in general. It also speaks to the importance of not assuming that groups do not change and highlights the dynamic state within which all groups are situated.

Menstruation

Most of the women whom we interviewed for our study on sexuality and women's health said that, as girls, they were given no explanation about the physical or emotional changes of puberty. One woman said, "I was nine years old when a friend told me that women were bleeding. I was scared. I walked around for three years just wondering and scaring myself [about] what it would be like. No explanation was made, just that I would bleed."

Women who had not been informed about menstruation were frightened when they bled for the first time: they thought they were dying. However, their fears were allayed when they asked their mothers for assistance and were told that this was a normal occurrence for women.

Some women had been forewarned about menstruation by their mother or an older sister. In all cases, however, only minimal information was transmitted: girls might be told that their period would occur monthly and was a private matter, and they might be advised about the necessary supplies. One reason for the lack of details was the poor understanding of female anatomy and physiology in the community as a whole. Menstrual periods were sometimes explained as a cleaning of the womb; one participant believed that menstrual blood was the foundation for a baby that had not been conceived. Another said that the period occurred after the eggs were released and travelled to the uterus. Even after decades of menstruation, interviewees had a limited understanding of why it occurred.

One woman told us that she was happy her girls were going to school and could read English because they brought home library books that illustrated female anatomy. Thanks to these books, she had finally begun to understand how her body worked and why menstruation occurred. For many women whom we interviewed, learning about this subject had been incidental, although the Mennonite lady doctor purposefully read and educated herself about topics that would aid her practice.

If women had difficult periods, they spoke with their mother. Some mothers suggested pain relievers that were easily purchased over the counter in a Mennonite pharmacia in Mexico or took their daughters to consult the Mennonite "doctor" in Mexico or Canada, who would prescribe what she saw as appropriate. Women commonly resorted to alternative treatments and often had non-scientific explanations for symptoms. For example, one woman who was unable to conceive until she migrated to Canada felt that the move had cured her infertility.

Reproduction

Regardless of their birthplace (Belize, Mexico, or Canada), most female interviewees had received little or no information about sexual intercourse. Children were seen as gifts from God, though more detailed discussion of their genesis did occur in some homes. A few individuals read books on sexuality that they found in Mexican bookstores, and one couple read such a book before they married. No interviewee had sought out similar material in Canada. Despite this lack of information and general reticence about sexuality, respondents did speak about sexual pleasure and their expectation that their husband would help them fulfill their desires.

Birth Control

Childbearing is central to the lives of LG Mennonite women. Historically, Mennonite families produced many children, which participants said was based on the directive that "you need to have as many children as God wants you to have." Scripture also supported fecundity: Psalm 127:3, for example, says, "Sons are indeed a heritage from the Lord, the fruit of the womb a reward."

In more than one study that I conducted, participants said that if a woman used birth control or aborted a fetus, the souls of her unborn children would wait at the gates of heaven to prevent her entry. It was therefore unsurprising to learn that few couples attempted to stagger the birth of their children or prevent pregnancy. Scripture states that, as long as a woman is faithful and acts in a spiritually sound manner, she will be cared for no matter how many children she has. Specifically, 1 Timothy 2:15 notes, "Yet she will be saved through child-bearing, provided they continue in faith and love and holiness, with modesty." Although interviewees generally said that they obeyed the dictates of their faith and did not use birth control, some had considered reducing their number of pregnancies. Even the Mennonite lady doctor, who believed that women should have as many children as God willed, admitted to prescribing birth control pills and intrauterine devices. The women knew that having more children would simply add to their workload and that their lives, particularly in Mexico, would always be difficult. They understood that they could not continue to give birth so frequently, and even when the husband did not agree, some took the chance of using birth control. One woman related that when her husband discovered her contraceptive equipment, he threw it out and told her that it was "a sin to use birth control." The women did worry about committing this sin. One told us that "using a condom did not feel quite as much as committing a sin [compared to other products]."

Only four of the thirty-eight women in the study on female sexuality had not used some form of birth control either in Mexico or Belize or since arriving in Canada. Although interviewees explained that they were expected to have as many children as God decreed, some opted for contraception. In some cases, a Mennonite "doctor" or a physician in Canada had suggested that they take a break from childbirth because of the stressfulness of their family life, an approach that helped husbands to accept family planning measures. According to one woman, her Mexican physician had told her that her "uterus is sick and needed to heal" as a way to justify the use of an injectable monthly contraceptive; another who used birth control said she had done so because she had "too much to carry," referring to emotional and physical hardships. The LG Mennonite liaison workers told us that, between 2003 and 2008, only a few members of this population had used birth control, but attitudes had shifted and it was now more common, especially among young couples. This was often a joint decision and was based on economic realities; the couple simply could not afford to raise the number of children that their parents had.

Our studies showed that when birth control was used, the severity of its side effects, ease of application, and cost determined which kind was chosen. Women referred to "monthly injections," probably of Depo Provera; in Mexico, these were obtained from physicians or purchased over the counter. Condoms were relatively cheap, and of course the rhythm method and withdrawal cost nothing at all. Although the women were familiar with these, they did not fully understand how they worked. Condoms were believed to prevent "the male stuff from getting in." Women who relied on the rhythm method kept track of their cycles to determine when they were fertile, but they employed a variety of counting systems. One woman said, "I found out after I got married that we menstruate to be able to have babies. I was very regular with my periods after I got married. I could have counted days if I had known about them." Some women referred to being more "open" on certain days of the month but could not always pinpoint when that was. Others were more specific, suggesting that intercourse was safe four days after the menstrual period. Another noted correctly that fifteen days afterward was not a safe time for unprotected intercourse.

Certain birth control methods were seen as unacceptable due to their permanency or side effects. For example, though some women had had tubal ligations, others said that the permanence of this measure made it inappropriate. Some cited its side effects; following a tubal ligation, some had experienced more painful periods or excessive clots. According to our respondents, the condom was the sole form of contraception available to men. When we asked about vasectomies, some replied that they had heard the procedure caused weight gain and reduced sexual desire.

Termination of Pregnancy

Unsurprisingly, birth control was a delicate topic, and our research assistants were careful to make the women feel safe in disclosing personal information. It was also the topic on which the norms of the women's social context had the greatest impact. Their most sensitive disclosure related to therapeutic or elective abortion. Some interviewees said that their physician had suggested a therapeutic abortion *(ursache felgeburt/ abtreiben)* to safeguard their health. However, they saw this as a radical departure from the teachings of the Bible and the church. In some communities, having a therapeutic abortion or even being suspected of doing so could potentially lead to excommunication and shunning. At the very least, it would signify to others that a woman had not followed the dictates of her church. Conforming to expected behaviours was always crucial because setting oneself apart could lead to divisiveness.

When the topic of abortion arose, our female interviewees always said that they had "heard that other women" had performed a folk abortion to terminate a pregnancy. We can only conclude that these women were driven by desperation. Some were young and unmarried, fully aware that neither their family nor their community would accept an illegitimate pregnancy. Some were in abusive and difficult marriages or were simply living intolerable lives with no emotional support. And some had already borne a number of children and felt physically or emotionally unprepared for more. Those who belonged to certain conservative churches could not count on church leaders for support and might decide to take matters into their own hands.

The women explained how to produce a miscarriage. It became apparent that "having a miscarriage" was their euphemism for "causing the baby to abort." Strategies included smelling bleach or other strong fumes such as vinegar or paint, jumping from apple trees, or drinking a mixture of wine in which rusty nails had been soaked.

In Belize, LG Mennonites focused on having what they called "regular periods." If their period were late, they injected each other with a hormone purchased over the counter in a local pharmacia. Although we cannot be certain, they may have been aborting early pregnancies consciously or unconsciously.

It is worth noting that the topic of folk abortions caused the greatest level of discomfort for the research advisory group – particularly its Mennonite members. This was not because they judged the women who had attempted to abort a fetus, but because they felt strong empathy for their situation and understood how difficult it must have been to take an action for which there was virtually no support.

Pregnancy and Childbirth

Being pregnant was referred to as *schwanger/droager* ("I am in a different time"), acknowledging the transition to an important physiological event. Being pregnant was highly private; the news was disclosed to the woman's mother and sisters, her husband and his mother, and close female friends. On some occasions, family members realized that a woman was expecting even before she did, which again indicates women's limited knowledge about their anatomy and physiology. Once she realized that she was pregnant, a woman focused all her physical, emotional, and spiritual energy on caring for herself and her unborn child. One woman said, "I think after three months the baby starts to live. It was alive after it started to move. The mom has to be careful through her whole pregnancy; something could happen to the baby at any time, because it's in her body the whole time."

Prenatal care during the early months of pregnancy was not common in Mexico and Belize, and even women who moved to Canada in the 1990s typically did not seek it out. However, whether they lived in Canada or Mexico, they did avoid certain activities to help ensure a healthy baby. These included heavy lifting, reaching up high (which might break the umbilical cord), crawling through barbed wire fences (which might wrap the cord around the baby's neck), using paints and strong cleaners (whose fumes could cause a miscarriage), eating spicy foods (which could harm the fetus), ingesting nerve pills and alcohol, and smoking cigarettes. Additionally, women were strongly encouraged to "clean their hearts" in preparation for a successful delivery.

Those who did not comply with the list of cautions were warned about either specific adverse results or the less defined prospect of having a sickly baby. The babies of those who drank would be slow to learn, and some interviewees in Canada also believed that an alcoholic father could negatively affect the fetus: because alcohol weakened his sperm, the newborn would have health problems.

According to interviewees, some behaviours that lay within the mother's control could affect the health of the baby. For example, a woman who did not atone for her sins would deliver a weak child, but it would gain strength if she sought spiritual guidance. Other influences on fetal health were beyond the control of the mother. Some unhealthy babies were simply the result of God's will and part of his plan. Certain incidents, such as a frightening experience, would produce an unhealthy baby or a birthmark. We were told about one woman who had been frightened by a snake and had placed her hand on her cheek; this imprint became a birthmark on the baby.

Extreme stress during pregnancy, including the death of a family member and its associated grief, and being unwell, were seen as linked with miscarriages. The mental state of the woman, especially her level of anxiety, was also thought to produce a miscarriage. In some instances, miscarriage could occur even if the woman avoided or undertook certain activities to prevent it. Interviewees believed that certain children were not meant to be born, because they had an illness of some type – in some cases due to genetic predisposition (which they described as "being in the blood"). Other reasons were that the uterus was "sick," the baby had not been "received right," was incorrectly attached to the cord and was thus not receiving adequate nutrition, or had died in the womb. Industrial chemicals from the fields were also blamed for causing miscarriages. In fact, this was not unlikely, given the agricultural work conducted by the men and the use of chemicals in some countries including Belize that are restricted in Canada. A pregnant woman who handled and washed the men's clothing could inadvertently ingest these toxins.

The pregnant woman and her husband were encouraged to engage in certain activities to help produce a healthy child. One of the most common was "turning the baby," which was seen as important because it would improve the comfort level of the mother and put the baby in the right position for an easy labour and delivery. Expectant mothers visited lay practitioners such as Mennonite "midwives" or "chiropractors" who turned the baby. To achieve this, the practitioner massaged the woman's abdomen so that the baby would turn itself and be head down. One woman talked about her experiences: "I was expected to go to a local midwife to have my babies turned. My mother told me that that's the thing I had to do, and the only time I went to a real doctor was when I was really sick."

A future mother was expected to eat a healthy diet, part of which included gratifying cravings. Failing to do so could produce a miscarriage or a weak baby, but opinions differed regarding alcohol consumption during pregnancy. One woman said,

> A woman should eat whatever she craves because that is what the baby needs, and if a woman craves beer or wine, that is okay, because that is what the baby needs and you should have it. And if there's anything you crave and you eat it or drink it, it will not affect the baby.

However, another woman said,

> I learned that the woman should eat what she craves because it can harm the baby if she doesn't. I never craved beer or wine. I don't drink that. I don't like it if women drink beer when they are pregnant. It's just not necessary. You hear that adults shouldn't drink, why would you give babies liquor? I don't know if the baby gets the alcohol that the mother drinks, but I think it is wrong.

Though their opinions differed, neither of these women fully understood how the body operates and how a pregnant woman is linked to a fetus. This lack of information can be ascribed to the family and community system in which they were raised and the greater social, historical, and political system that informed their lives.

A pregnant woman was required to follow her mother's suggestions in taking care of herself and to obey the advice of the lay practitioners or Mexican or Canadian physicians whom she saw. In the provinces where we conducted our research, translators or LG Mennonite liaison workers helped women to access care from formal practitioners such as physicians or public health nurses. Sometimes Mennonite women preferred that the boundaries between alternative and formal practitioners be blurred rather than defined. As a case in point, one woman said,

> In my fourth pregnancy, I had a difficult labour because the baby was turned the wrong way. The nurses told me to walk lots, but I wanted the Mennonite chiropractor lady to come to the hospital but the nurses refused. I went outside for a walk with my husband and visited the Mennonite chiropractor around the corner, so that she could turn the baby. One hour later the baby was born.

We interviewed a Mennonite woman who was referred to as a "lady doctor." This self-trained individual said that when she practised in Mexico, she required all expectant mothers to have an ultrasound at seven months to prevent difficulties in labour. She requested that those with a breech presentation be delivered by a Mexican physician.

Once a woman went into labour, she anticipated a normal delivery if she had followed the guidelines described above. Difficult births were attributed to the baby being turned the wrong way, but no delivery was expected to be free of discomfort. This too was traced to the Bible. According to Genesis 3:16, when God punished Eve for her transgression in the Garden of Eden, he said, "I will greatly increase your pangs in childbearing; in pain you shall bring forth children, yet your desire shall be for your husband, and he shall rule over you."

All women were subject to this penalty. Thus, by God's decree, childbirth automatically involved pain.

Postpartum Health

After delivery, the new mother and baby received substantial support from female relatives and friends, who prepared meals for the woman and her family for up to six weeks. In some instances, the new mother's younger sisters moved into her home and helped with the chores. Some women told us that they had very supportive husbands, who relieved them of their normal tasks, such as milking the cows, for the first six weeks after a baby was born. Beyond avoiding hard work and resting in the early stage of postpartum, the woman's only restriction was to avoid foods that would cause discomfort to her or the baby.

The interviewees noted that baby blues were common, but their descriptions revealed that they were more probably referring to postpartum depression. (Baby blues are mood swings and crying spells that occur for a short time after birth, whereas postpartum depression is a more severe form of depression that can last for several months. Some women experience postpartum psychosis, a serious mental illness that should be treated as a medical emergency.) Twenty-four of the thirty-eight women who participated in the study on women's health and sexuality were specifically asked about postpartum depression, and thirteen said they had experienced it. For the majority, feelings of sadness and being overwhelmed were fleeting, but one recalled that she had been extremely depressed and had even desired to "be in heaven" – a wish she had not acted upon. The LG Mennonite liaison workers voiced their concerns regarding the prevalence of postpartum depression, a not infrequent complaint within their communities, and noted that women also asked for "nerve pills" when they visited a Canadian physician. We had no precise information regarding these pills, but they were probably intended to strengthen the nerves, a topic that will be examined in Chapter 5.

We discussed breastfeeding with interviewees. A number said that their milk was watery and too weak, so they relied on store-bought formula. As was the case with other physiological conditions, they believed that engaging in certain activities would increase or diminish the production of breast milk. Some felt that beer drinking would increase it, though the effects on the baby were unknown. Just as when they were pregnant, women were advised to avoid specific activities, such as cleaning or painting, because hard work would stop milk production.

Other Health Issues

During our interviews, we also asked women about any surgeries they may have had. They reported that hysterectomies did occur, though for the more conservative LG Mennonites, this decision required a discussion with the woman's husband and her minister. Importantly, the women referred to a hysterectomy as "Das life eruet naemen," which translates to "taking the mother out." This word choice reflects the nature of their roles in the Mennonite community.

Throughout our years of interviewing women, we met a number who did not receive adequate support from their communities in Canada. In one case, a woman and her family had left a conservative church and moved to a more liberal one because the former had often failed to support the family or display interest in it. In some situations, community members sided with the ministers and did not question their treatment of certain families.

If a woman experienced mental health problems such as depression, she might not receive community support. Some ministers and lay people saw depression as shameful and could merely dismiss the woman as lazy, declining to consider any alternative explanation for her state of mind. Rumours would circulate about her, and she would receive no offers of assistance.

Our interviewees showed additional facets to suffering. For example, a woman who had experienced a miscarriage could find comfort in the belief that God had taken the child because it was ill and would not allow it to suffer on earth. The miscarriage could help her to place her trust in God. Women who had multiple miscarriages would be forced to reflect on their own spiritual behaviour to determine whether changes were required. As previously mentioned, it was believed that women who did not atone for their sins would deliver children with health problems. Those who chose to smoke and drink, and generally to stray from God, would reap the consequences when they gave birth.

Interviewees believed that suffering and difficult circumstances were a test from God. One woman whose child was disabled said, "I just think that this is a cross that I have to carry, and you do just that." Another said, "We are expected to suffer so that we will trust God and [because we receive] his help." This is reinforced by Mark 9:23: "If you are able! – All things can be done for the one who believes." For the women, assisting others who were suffering was also a way of pleasing God and demonstrating moral goodness.

Domestic Violence

Women were expected to care for others, but some felt that they themselves were not cared for or supported by their churches or communities. Several women, including victims of domestic violence, told us they felt abandoned by their community. This was not entirely surprising, because some Mennonite churches see women as the ultimate cause of spousal abuse.

We gained first-hand experience of this attitude in 2001, when the Southern Alberta Kanadier Association (SAKA) committee, of which I was a member, began to conduct community development projects. We wanted to address sensitive issues such as domestic violence, as we had reliable evidence from the Mennonite liaison worker that it was a problem in the community. Hoping to collaborate with all churches simultaneously, we attempted to arrange a meeting with the leadership of the four largest churches in southern Alberta, but this proved problematic. Only one church was willing to meet with the others, so we had to meet four separate times with the leadership of each church. In addition, we had to ensure that a male SAKA member was present at every meeting; if he were not there, the ministers would be disinclined to attend or answer our questions.

The meeting with the most conservative church was held at a public health office. The bishop, ministers, deacon, and their respective wives came as a group to discuss our questions. One of the SAKA members was a Mennonite liaison worker who was fluent in Plautdietsch and was thus able to provide translation during the meeting. All of our questions needed to be filtered through the male member of SAKA. Our agenda moved from the less delicate topics to those of greater sensitivity. Our spokesman cautiously asked about domestic violence and how it could be addressed within the community. As the bishop responded at length in Plautdietsch, the liaison worker's expression became increasingly exasperated. When he finally stopped speaking, she said to us, "Basically, he said that if a woman is abused by her husband, she deserves it, because she probably burnt the supper or something like that." We all sat in silence. The difficulty of diminishing domestic violence was now obvious to us, and we understood how little support there was for women.

We learned that, despite this general belief, women themselves did not feel they had to accept spousal abuse. It was not a cross that they needed to bear. One participant said that she was subjected to domestic violence and that her husband had sexually abused their two daughters, with the result that each had given birth to one child. She received no support from her community in Mexico and, in desperation, decided to drown herself in a lake. However, when she attempted to do so, a white light appeared to her. Interpreting this as a sign from God, she returned to her family. Soon afterward, they moved to Canada and through a variety of circumstances, her husband was removed from the home and placed in jail.

In LG Mennonite communities, women's health is rooted in their religious beliefs and informed by the expectations of community members as well as their social, economic, historical, and political context. Due to the sensitive nature of the topic, female anatomy and physiology are not well understood by LG Mennonites and tend not to be openly discussed. In addition, depending upon their particular circumstances and community, women may not receive support when they experience domestic violence or mental health problems. The religious beliefs of the group govern expectations regarding family size and the acceptability of birth control. Simultaneously, women play a significant role in caring for their family members or the wider community, thereby contributing to general well-being. Finally, LG Mennonites display significant strength in dealing with challenging circumstances and typically rely on faith to cope with suffering.

4

DEATH AND DYING

Low German Mennonite beliefs and practices related to death and dying are steeped in tradition, which provides comfort and support to community members. The purpose of our formal study on this topic was not only to gain an understanding of it, but also to develop care guidelines for health practitioners, social workers, and non-Mennonite ministers. We conducted interviews in Alberta and Manitoba (Kulig & Fan, 2013a, 2013b, 2013c), and additional fieldwork in Durango Colony, Mexico. The LG Mennonites who participated in the study represented a range of churches, from conservative to liberal.

We interviewed fifty-eight LG Mennonites (twenty-five males and thirty-three females) in Alberta and Manitoba but derived additional information from other studies in the research program, including fifteen additional interviews in Mexico. The participants ranged in age from twenty-one to eighty-four and had a variety of experiences caring for relatives who had died; some were facing the death of a friend or family member. Their views are based on their experiences in Canada, Mexico, Belize, and Bolivia. The findings discussed here focus on beliefs and practices in Canada but, where applicable, examples are provided that illustrate an experience in these other locales.

Views on Death and Dying

Religious doctrine is ingrained in LG Mennonite beliefs related to death and dying. Very little literature deals with LG Mennonite views on this important life transition, so our study filled a major gap in the understanding of the community's perspectives, illustrating the complex relationship between spiritual beliefs and practices related to death.

During her fieldwork in Chihuahua, Kerstin Reinschmidt (2001) found that LG Mennonites see life as uncertain and thus believe they must be prepared to meet death at all times. Mennonites who believe in God believe that eternal life begins with death. They understand that a key step in achieving eternal salvation is to live in a way that prepares them for death. One way of preparing is to give to others, a basic tenet of their religion. At the foundation of their beliefs is a commitment to follow God's word and learn forgiveness. Their pledge to help others and to work hard helps fulfill that duty.

The LG Mennonite participants in all our research projects expressed similar beliefs about death. Because God alone determined when death would come, it was important to be ready for dying. They freely discussed the requirement to help others as a way of preparing for a meaningful death. Adults needed to be spiritually healthy, which meant that God must be present in their heart and that they must shun the temptations of Satan. One participant said, "A person who invites Jesus into his life, asks for forgiveness, and seeks to live a life that is pleasing to God is one who is prepared to meet God when he dies." Individuals who die suddenly but who give to others and are spiritually healthy on an ongoing basis will be prepared to face God.

Since no one can know how others feel in their hearts – in other words, no one can be sure that another person is spiritually healthy – LG Mennonites are uncertain about the fate of those who die suddenly. If community members lose a relative unexpectedly – in a car accident, for example – they worry that the victim may not have had time to prepare to meet God.

The family unit plays an integral role in caring for infirm and dying individuals, regardless of their age or gender. The women provide physical care and prayer, asking God to intervene or comfort the ill or dying person. Men are the decision makers with respect to care.

Some families prefer that a relative die in hospital rather than at home, so that the physician "can help until the end," as one participant put it. Some LG Mennonites believe that God directs the end-of-life care provided by the physician. One interviewee expanded on this belief and offered another reason for choosing hospitalization:

> I prefer a person to die in the hospital or nursing home, because they can give better care and help to make it easier for the dying person. The other reason why I prefer a person to not die at home is that sometimes that room where a person dies stays too much in the mind of the other family members. Some get scared at night. I know [of] one lady who moved into another bedroom from where her husband had died.

It is worth noting that decisions regarding the care of elderly or terminally ill individuals, particularly parents, often fall to the eldest son, who speaks with the physician and then consults with his minister. On the whole, the opinions of physicians concerning treatment, surgery, and palliative care are highly respected, and the family normally abides by them once the son makes his decision.

Interviewees said they were willing to receive care from both male and female non-Mennonite providers such as nurses and physicians, though they preferred them to be Christians. One participant said that health providers "make the person comfortable, wash and feed them. Some of the nurses will give good spiritual care as well, like reading Bible verses [and doing other things to] comfort them."

Another reinforced this sentiment by saying that providers needed to "care for [patients] in a Christ-like manner."

LG Mennonites who are informed by their physician that death is imminent know that they must "set [their] house in order," as counselled by Isaiah 38:1. For baptized adults, this entails ensuring that they are spiritually healthy, which includes atoning for their sins – acknowledging their offences and asking for forgiveness. One participant said, "Preparing for death means that a person would take time to pray, ask for forgiveness from people and from God, and receive peace with everyone. It also includes clarifying things with the bank account and other arrangements." Another interviewee said that the dying must "search the well-being of their soul, make up a will, teach their family all they can while they can."

The most common message from participants was that the dying must formally ask forgiveness from anyone whom they had wronged or hurt. They must also forgive those who had injured them. Reconciling their relationships with others strengthened their ties with God. Spending time with their minister helped them to acknowledge the imperfections of their life on earth and to change their behaviour. By praying with them and urging them to atone for their sins and seek the forgiveness of others, the minister aided their efforts to put their spiritual health in order and to prepare for their journey to the afterlife.

When someone was dying, the family expected frequent visits from ministers, who could come by unannounced to spend time with the individual and the family. As a result, the patient's room could become quite crowded. This style of visiting was seen as crucial to the dying person's well-being. Particularly when death was imminent, people often wished simply to "be" with a dying relative, quietly sitting with him so that he would not be alone. "Being with" could also include singing hymns to comfort family members as they died.

Close relatives and friends spent time in prayer with dying individuals, with whom they could exchange forgiveness. This process of atonement was so essential that interviewees openly voiced their preference for a slow death rather than a quick one, because it enabled them to make amends for their sins and forgive others. One participant said, "I prefer a period of time [to die] because it gives the dying person a chance to prepare for death. But sometimes the Devil will try to make people doubt about their faith, and that is very hard." Another said, "Prepare for death, to let go of the people close to the dying person and also their belongings and surroundings, discuss issues of life and make suggestions to ... those who will be surviving, and just get things right with everybody around them and also with God." Some LG Mennonites view angels as a tangible presence that helps them address their needs when they are ill; however, this topic was not commonly discussed by the participants.

Some LG Mennonites practise the laying on of hands, placing hands on the sick or dying while praying. They also apply blessed water to the foreheads of those who are near death. Both of these rituals are conducted by women. Anointing with water may be seen as lying outside a minister's purview, so community members perform it. There is some indication in the literature that anointing includes the use of oil to bless the sick (Wenger, 2000). Originally, this was not part of a minister's duties, but it has been gradually accepted by some Mennonite churches and can be fully performed using oil (Wenger, 2000).

Chapter 3 highlighted that suffering is a common theme in the research on LG Mennonites; our study on death and dying reinforced this fact. Interviewees discussed both physical and spiritual suffering but tended to concentrate on the latter. Generally speaking, suffering was seen as beneficial because it enabled individuals to restore their connection with God and to receive forgiveness for their sins. Death constituted a release from suffering if they had genuinely atoned for their sins and developed a positive relationship with God.

Palliative Care and End-of-Life Measures

Our interviewees shared their opinions of palliative care, including end-of-life directives. Many criticized palliative care as an admission that there was "no hope" for a sick individual and that death was being allowed to occur (Fan, 2011). They did not see it as a compassionate service for people who had contracted a serious and probably terminal illness. It is also difficult to translate "palliative care" into Plautdietsch so that it can be fully understood. A number of participants said they would not accept care for a relative if it were formally called "palliative" or if it involved placing the person in a room that was set aside for palliative care. They saw this approach as hastening death. The health care professionals with whom we spoke understood that LG Mennonites would not easily accept palliative care. In fact, it was at odds with their beliefs – because God alone determined when a person would die, accepting palliative care did not acknowledge his ability to alter the life course of an individual.

End-of-life directives are written documents that instruct family members regarding the care of relatives who can no longer make their own decisions. Most interviewees felt that such documents were unacceptable. Once again, they emphasized that God alone chose the moment of death; thus, setting up care guidelines for an individual whom medical science had identified as terminal would be presumptuous. Decisions about administering cardiopulmonary resuscitation (CPR), for instance, would be made if and when it were required, rather than in advance. Should CPR fail to work, it was because God had decided that the person would die. To reinforce this, participants mentioned that "God does not make mistakes"; in other words, he knew all and made the correct decisions regarding life and death.

In addition, some interviewees preferred to give oral instructions to key relatives that could be followed when necessary. Although this illustrates the manner in which LG Mennonites make decisions, it reflects an unawareness that during a crisis, when immediate action is essential, relying on oral directions may simply prove unworkable. It also reveals lack of understanding that oral instructions do not satisfy the legalities governing consent in the provision of health care.

"Life support" includes a range of activities and technologies to extend a person's life. Depending on the gravity of the condition, it may not be useful, but if it were offered to an LG Mennonite, the family would need to consult with their minister. LG Mennonites are familiar with the concept of "brain death," but their approach to it may differ markedly from that of health providers. From their religious point of view, there is always hope that an individual will recover. In fact, several participants related incidents in which comatose people who were not expected to live not only regained consciousness but also experienced a full recovery. One interviewee shared the story of a brother-in-law who had been in a coma; after a week, the physician had given up hope of his recovery, but the family wanted to wait and give him more time. After three weeks, he regained consciousness and spoke about his experience of being in a coma. This example highlighted God's merciful power, which allowed the man to revive.

Interviewees cited an additional and more serious reservation about life support – whether its removal would hasten death. This concern applied even to brain-dead patients who had no hope of recovery. Ministers and lay people discussed this topic at great length and were very concerned that their decision or advice to a family might bring about the death of an individual. From a religious perspective, if death were accelerated by the removal of life support, it would be euthanasia – a practice that LG Mennonites unequivocally oppose. Some ministers talked candidly about the dilemma of advising families who asked about discontinuing life support. They wanted the dying individual to receive optimal care but also wanted to assure the family that their decision coincided with the principles of the faith. This highlights the LG Mennonite focus on integrating spiritual and physical health, and the conviction that both must be addressed.

Death and Burial

When a community member dies, the minister is called to the home or facility to provide support for the family and prayers for the deceased. LG Mennonites do not engage in organ donation, because organs that are viable for transplant must still be "alive." For LG Mennonites, this infers that the donor is not dead. None of our interviewees favoured cremation, because of their belief that the corpse must decompose and return to dust.

Before the funeral, the body must be prepared for burial. In Mexico and Belize, certain women in the community performed this important task. I interviewed one woman who had learned it from her mother and had then offered the service for decades in her village in Durango Colony, Mexico. She was available at all times of the day and night, and had a kit of materials and supplies standing ready. Over the years, she had tended to people who had died in a variety of ways, including naturally, accidentally, and by suicide. Family members sometimes helped her prepare the body. Her work was an integral part of community life.

The involvement of community members in digging the grave and participating in the burial varies by geographic location. Some LG Mennonites in Canada still dig graves by hand. Generally, a number of LG Mennonites act as pallbearers and place the casket in the ground themselves, rather than relying on funeral staff to do so. Family members are not routinely buried next to each other, as the choice of where to dig a grave is determined by the space available in the cemetery rather than the desire of relatives to lie close together.

Funerals

Participants were divided on the question of whether children should go to funerals. At a funeral I attended in Mexico, the immediate relatives of the deceased all brought their children; friends of the children of the deceased, who were between the ages of four and twenty, also attended. However, some of our Bolivian participants noted that only children of close family members went to funerals in that country. One Bolivian interviewee said that children were excluded from the funerals of women who had died in childbirth; she attributed this restriction to the emphasis of conservative churches on shielding children from distressing realities, such as the fact that women can die in childbirth. In Canada, unless children were closely related to the deceased, they were not always taken out of school to attend a funeral. In general, however, they were not discouraged from going, because funerals enabled them to support the grieving family while respecting the deceased. In addition, funerals conveyed valuable lessons about living in a spiritually healthy manner.

Depending upon the church, the funeral service could indicate whether the deceased had followed God's path or had atoned for sins and received forgiveness. It reflected his or her spirituality and choice to live as God directed. Interviewees mentioned various aspects of the service, including the singing of hymns, a sermon regarding the Christian behaviour of the deceased, a community viewing of the body, and the interment of the casket.

When we attempted to discuss the afterlife with participants, we found that many were uncomfortable with talking about it, saying that "they had not been there yet." Others expected that it would be wonderful because it involved spending eternity with Jesus. Salvation was a dominant theme, but perspectives varied according to church affiliation. Members of conservative churches did not automatically assume that they would go to heaven, even if their faith were strong. Members of more liberal churches agreed that having faith in God and in Christ was essential to securing a place in heaven. Regardless of their church, participants felt that salvation was determined by God's judgment; the sinful would find it difficult to enter heaven. Mennonite scholars have discussed the theological differences between churches' views of salvation (see, for example, Quiring, 1997).

Unconventional Burials

Reinschmidt (2001) notes that LG Mennonite funerals remind the family of the deceased that they are not alone and that the community shares in their loss. Although this generally holds true, our interviews revealed that it was not always the case. In certain circumstances, families could feel that a funeral did not provide the support they needed at the time of such significant loss. Interviewees commonly mentioned two examples of such funerals: for excommunicants and those who had died by suicide.

An individual could be excommunicated for a variety of reasons, including engaging in a lifestyle that deviated from the principles of the church. Alcoholics and those who used illegal drugs or abused prescription medication ran the risk of being excommunicated, as did adulterers or those who physically or sexually abused their children. The funeral service for an excommunicant could depart from the norm, depending upon the decision of the minister. The deceased could be referred to as a friend rather than a brother or sister, and the body might be displayed outside the church rather than within it. The sermon could highlight the errant behaviour of the deceased as a way of instructing listeners on how to behave. Excommunicants who attended the funeral of a relative might not be permitted to sit with the family or might have to sit in another room; at the *faspa,* a post-funeral luncheon at which coffee and baked goods are provided to community members, they might be forced to sit with the children.

No Mennonite church condones suicide. However, among the conservative churches, particularly those in Mexico, suicide is considered even more unfavourable to the individual and his or her family than it is in liberal churches. As with excommunicants, funerals and burials of those who die by suicide may diverge from the norm. During the funeral, the body may be placed outside the church or building. We were told of individuals who were buried a foot deeper than usual as punishment for having killed themselves, a measure that would move them one foot closer to hell. Some ministers believed that people who died by suicide were "going straight to hell"; there was little consideration of the challenges they might have faced, the difficulties of their lives, or how the lack of understanding or support from the church might have affected them. We were told that some people who died by suicide were buried outside the cemetery or in a corner away from the other graves (a practice that also occurs in some mainstream Canadian churches). Most importantly, instead of being positioned so that their feet pointed to the east, they would be rotated to face west. This guaranteed that they would not connect with God, because they could not rise up and meet him during the Second Coming.

The relatives of an LG Mennonite who dies by suicide are left with the knowledge that he or she has been buried in the "wrong" direction and has thus been denied rising up with God. They must contend with the realization that his or her eternal salvation is now in jeopardy, while simultaneously grieving their loss and coming to terms with the manner of the relative's death.

For LG Mennonites, the lifestyle choices and circumstances of others provide lessons on living in a spiritually healthy way, which ultimately enhances the community's spiritual strength. Learning about the transgressions of those who have died, such as infidelity, substance abuse, or suicide, teaches community members about the consequences of behaviour that is not tolerated by the church. We were given many examples of ministers who delivered stern lectures during funerals to emphasize the poor choices of the deceased and how those choices had resulted in death. In Mexico, we were told of an LG Mennonite man who was driving while intoxicated and became involved in a car accident that killed his spouse and children. He was brought from the hospital by stretcher to attend their funeral. During the sermon, the minister publicly admonished him and stated that he was to blame for their deaths. LG Mennonites believe that children who attend such funerals will hear the message and refrain from making bad choices.

Interviewees mentioned various other burial practices, such as the ritual interment of amputated body parts, which some ministers and communities accepted. For example, individuals who had lost a limb due to diabetes could have it formally buried. They typically prepared a box lined with fabric in which to place the body part. The minister was asked to come to the graveyard and assist with its burial, in a ceremony that was usually attended only by close family. It was not unusual for limbs to be buried in a grave that was already occupied by a relative, such as a parent. If amputees subsequently experienced phantom pain (the sensation of pain in a body part that is no longer there), they attributed it to the incorrect placement of the limb in the box and sometimes dug it up, adjusted the limb, and reinterred it.

Burials of Infants and Children

In some parts of Canada, a woman who miscarried or had a stillbirth would have the fetus buried in a grave occupied by another family member, rather than burying it alone. Sometimes, a local Mennonite approached the health care facility on her behalf, requesting that the fetus be surrendered for interment.

Interviewees, both lay and clerical, asserted that children born out of wedlock were not responsible for the indiscretions of their parents and would thus be buried in the regular manner, with their feet pointing east. One participant said, "Kids are accepted by God, no matter how they are conceived or born. It's not their fault if they come out of wedlock. Babies have souls, too. The Bible says, 'God says, I knew you when you were still in your mother's womb.'" An interviewee from Bolivia explained that the soul enters the child at the moment of conception, so all children possess a soul regardless of whether they are illegitimate. Another participant supported these sentiments: "I just know that every baby, born or unborn, is a child of God and it [the baby] needs to be taken care of. To the mother, it [the miscarriage] is a loss. We once held a service for a four-month-old fetus that was miscarried." During her fieldwork in Cuauhtémoc, Mexico, LingLing Fan located a cemetery that was devoted exclusively to children and babies. One grave was rotated from the usual direction, so that the child's feet pointed west. We showed a photo of the grave to a number of ministers and other individuals, all of whom were surprised. None could explain why the child had been buried in this way.

Supporting Those Left Behind

In Mexico and other southern locales, as well as in Canada, the community and the church provide support for a widow or widower, but it is not uncommon for remarriage to occur soon after the death of a spouse. In many cases, this is a practical decision given the onerousness of being a single parent. In Mexico, the Waisenamt – a committee within the Mennonite village that focuses on the social welfare of orphans, widows, and widowers – is tasked with protecting the social interests of children and will ask the surviving parent to select a mentor or guide who will provide advice that will assist in raising the children. If the mentor is the mother, she will be asked to assign a mentor for herself. If the parents of underage children both die simultaneously, the Waisenamt discusses the circumstances of the orphans and decides what will happen to them. It determines whether the children will be kept together in one home or be separated and moved into individual homes in the community. In Canada, with its social services bureaucracy, making decisions about the living circumstances of orphaned minors is a legal matter. In Alberta, efforts have been made to set up foster homes that can care for LG Mennonite children. The foster families have either a Mennonite background or are sufficiently familiar with the group that they can help children cope with the loss of their family.

Among LG Mennonites, patterning one's life upon the teachings of Jesus by helping others and making appropriate choices in accordance with church doctrine is seen as essential to achieving eternal salvation. Even when death is imminent, one can always make amends for past transgressions, through the process of atonement. When a family member is dying, female relatives provide care, whereas the men – typically the father or the eldest son – make the necessary decisions to ease suffering. In such circumstances, families often rely on church teachings and the support of ministers. Funeral and burial practices vary from conservative to liberal churches, but all agree that even in death people can learn to live in a manner that pleases God. Health care providers must develop strategies that support and respect LG Mennonite religious beliefs and practices while simultaneously assisting individuals who are struggling with the decisions of their ministers regarding the treatment of relatives, both before and after death.

5
MENTAL HEALTH

Throughout our interviews with Low German Mennonites, participants frequently referred to mental health and its impact on their everyday lives. To enhance our understanding of this important topic, we launched a study that focused specifically on LG Mennonite beliefs regarding mental health. The present chapter is grounded in information gathered by this study (Kulig & Fan, 2016a, 2016b), which took place in Alberta, Manitoba, and Ontario, but also includes information gathered during fieldwork in Durango Colony, Mexico. The interviews from our other research studies also provided information about mental health and wellness, and relevant comments are included here. Unless otherwise noted, the chapter focuses on participants' lives in Canada. The ideas presented here are placed within the social context of LG Mennonite religious beliefs, highlighting variations based upon church affiliation.

We interviewed thirty-five LG Mennonites in Canada, nineteen females and sixteen males, who ranged in age from twenty-four to seventy-nine, as well as fifteen participants in Mexico. Participants were either mentally ill themselves or were caring for someone who was self-diagnosed or had been diagnosed with a mental illness by a health provider. Some were caring for a husband or wife who had schizophrenia or depression, or were struggling themselves with conditions such as postpartum depression. Their poignant comments illustrated their daily challenges and their reliance on their spiritual beliefs as a source of strength.

Previous Findings

There is little information and even less formal research that focuses on mental health and illness among LG Mennonites. According to some published sources, conservative LG Mennonites believe that mental illness should be addressed through the church and individual prayer rather than through more "worldly" ways (Quiring, 1997). In her research on women's health and illness in Mexico, Reinschmidt (2001) found that participants linked health to relationships among community members. They described narvenkrankheit a folk illness that is also called "sickness of nerves" or "weak nerves," as having a negative impact on these relationships. Narvenkrankheit produces inappropriate emotions and unusual behaviours, and results in psychosomatic symptoms. Reinschmidt's participants said that it could afflict both adults and children, and her respondents from conservative churches categorized a range of mental and emotional health issues, including misconduct and anti-social behaviour, as narvenkrankheit. Because LG Mennonites rely on harmonious interactions between family and community members, individuals who act inappropriately are disruptive to community life. Reinschmidt concluded that narvenkrankheit was probably the equivalent of depression and that it stemmed from problems with social relationships during childhood; her participants expected that people who had narvenkrankheit must learn to manage their "nerves." This involved the use of faith-based strategies, such as prayer, by both the individual and the wider community.

Reinschmidt (2001, p. 336) found that deviant behaviours – and, indeed, all personal problems – were seen as shameful and sinful. Shame, combined with a shortage of *Seelsorger* (ministers trained to address soul sickness), could lead to depression and even suicide. Finally, Reinschmidt's research revealed that gossip could be used as an instrument of social control, enforcing the community's moral norms and protecting it from behaviours that were seen as threatening to the group. For example, people who drank could become the focus of gossip that was intended to teach them the unacceptability of their behaviour and the need for change. However, not all community members appreciated this social pressure.

Diane Quadros (2009) discusses the experiences of LG Mennonite women with the provincial mental health services of Ontario. She asked six women about their definitions of mental health, their experiences with the provincial services, and their personal strategies in coping with the challenge of accessing them. She conducted her interviews in English. The six women were dealing with depression but none had been diagnosed with a psychotic condition. They described mental illness as having "nerves" or having "a breakdown." Having a breakdown meant no longer being able to control their symptoms and thus needing help from others, whether that be family, church, or physicians. A theme of the interviews was the need to keep their depression a secret from others, including their spouses. They hid their sadness in their "hearts," locked away inside themselves. They were not familiar with mental illness – as a concept or because they weren't aware of anyone who suffered from it – and could not recognize its signs and symptoms. They did not feel supported by their church or community.[1] In fact, the women, and sometimes their relatives, received telephone calls from community members that criticized their behaviour and instructed them to attend church more frequently to regain their health. In this community, the physically ill could ask for and receive help from others, but such was not the case if the problem were mental illness. The church was equally unsupportive when the women approached its leaders for assistance.

The six interviewees did talk positively about the care they received from their physicians; some also attended a community support group that was separate from their church group. Although they did use prescription medication to treat their symptoms, they also said that prayer was integral in helping them deal with their illness. Once their symptoms abated, family members questioned the continued use of their medication, revealing a failure to understand that mental illness is a disease rather than a controllable behaviour. The women reiterated that they did not often receive support from their family or the community. Finally, they described the submissive nature of their relationships with their husband, which included obeying his instructions that they not talk about their "nerve" problems with anyone else.

Mental and Spiritual Health and Illness

Our study found that LG Mennonites had difficulty discussing concepts such as health, mental health, mental illness, spiritual health, and spiritual illness. They described good mental health as being able to make decisions independently, which implied that an individual could think clearly, thereby making decisions that followed the word of God. Most participants differentiated between spiritual and mental wellness and illness but did see connections between the two. Respondents said that spiritual health began by developing a relationship with God that was maintained through reading Scripture, praying, and going to church. A basic aspect of spiritual wellness was entrusting their lives to God. Some noted that being spiritually well meant having a purpose in life; others stated that people who were spiritually well did not become discouraged when they encountered setbacks.

Participants identified spiritually strong people as those who could make sound choices that ensured good mental health. A person who did not believe in God was not spiritually well. Being spiritually and mentally well was helpful in overcoming depression. However, because studying Scripture and living by it were keys to spiritual health, interviewees from conservative churches were concerned about how to maintain it, as they were not permitted to read the Bible.

A number of interviewees could not identify specific reasons for a relative's mental illness. Among those who did, some felt that the individual could not control it, whereas others disagreed. This distinction is important because LG Mennonites often do not understand that mental illness cannot be managed by an act of will.

Of those who felt that a mental disorder was outside an individual's control, most attributed it to genetics. They described it as "running in the family." One stated that certain people were susceptible to "weak nerves" and to mental problems. Participants could not elaborate on this idea, except to refer to families that had a number of suicides and a range of mental issues. For example, a woman whom I interviewed in Durango Colony talked about her own relatives; some had died by suicide and some were prey to anxiety and panic attacks, but she could not explain why, beyond surmising that it was due to family traits.

Some respondents said that the mentally ill could not control their thoughts and emotions; they felt that mental disorders were related to the *vestaunt* (brain). A male participant said that, due to his experience with a brother who had schizophrenia, he believed that the mentally ill were not in touch with reality. As in the study on health and illness (Kulig et al., 2002), participants described being mentally unwell as having *narfun trubble* (nerve trouble) or "weak" or "bad" nerves. They also referred to people with mental health issues as *dvautsch* (crazy or different), and they cited unusual, anti-social, or "hidden" behaviours. The mentally ill could not help the way they felt – in other words, they had not chosen to be sick.

Stress was also believed to lead to mental illness, but respondents did not say whether an individual could take steps to avoid or reduce it. One stated that mental problems arose from a chemical imbalance, and a woman noted that they could be caused by war or experiencing a lack of respect. She also said that the mentally ill were angels on earth who needed to be treated kindly.

Some participants believed that if people were strong enough, they could overcome the potential to develop a mental disorder, which implied that mental illness was a choice. Older people were seen as more capable of dealing with difficulties because they had more life experience. There was some consensus that women were generally stronger than men and more able to cope with problems in their lives. Despite this perception, two phrases occurred repeatedly: "Men turn to drinking; women have nerves" and "Men get angry and violent; women stay in bed and cry."

Respondents said that being mentally unwell served a purpose: it could shed new light on the life of an individual while enhancing compassion for others who suffered. They emphasized the importance of not passing judgment on the mentally ill.

Some interviewees believed that all aspects of health and illness, including mental issues, emanated from God. The help required to deal with illness – including mental illness – was also God-given. Some believed that having a relative who was sick, whether physically or mentally, was "God willing difficulties as our cross to bear." One young woman had heard that "our punishments are laid out for us to endure on earth," noting that all human experiences were predetermined.

Participants discussed various types of mental illness, such as depression (which they saw as the most common mental problem among LG Mennonites), anxiety, bipolar disorder (which some referred to as manic depression), and schizophrenia (the most frequently mentioned psychotic condition). They felt that eating disorders such as bulimia were a kind of mental illness and were more common in women than in men. Everyone pointed out that women could have the baby blues; some referred specifically to postpartum depression and acknowledged its seriousness, but whether they understood the difference between the two conditions was not always clear. Some participants did not discuss postpartum depression to any great extent; a research assistant speculated that, because it was an aspect of women's health and was tied to sexuality, it was not openly discussed, especially not by men, who saw it as a woman's problem, not something they needed to know about. According to one interviewee, postpartum depression signalled that "nerves were low," and some believed that it was caused by a deficiency in folic acid or vitamins such as B12. Throughout our years of researching LG Mennonites, including in this study, we were often told that women with postpartum depression were lazy, again suggesting that being depressed was a matter of individual control.

When asked about how women with postpartum depression coped, participants replied that they were sometimes unable to care for their children and thus needed help from others. One stated that the mother should "keep trying" to care for the baby, once again implying that the condition was controllable. In extreme cases, the mother could die by suicide or resort to infanticide. Daily prayer and reliance on God were seen as crucial in dealing with the situation. Medications and counselling were also mentioned as important aspects of care.

Shame, Sin, and Suffering

Shame, sin, and suffering play a key role in shaping LG Mennonite beliefs about mental health. The family can be deeply ashamed of having a relative who is mentally unwell. They realize that community members will gossip about them and judge them rather than provide support. The fear of gossip exacerbates the tendency to hide mental illness from view. To avoid becoming the subject of gossip, people keep their troubles to themselves, which simply worsens stress for mentally ill individuals and the relatives who are trying to help them. Our participants felt that most church leaders and community members had no understanding of mental illness or its symptoms. One example mentioned was of a mentally ill man who had acted inappropriately in church, debating the interpretation of the Bible with the ministers – something unheard of in conservative churches. He also destroyed household objects with an axe and threw them out of his home in full sight of the neighbours. In the LG Mennonite community, as in the rest of the world, keeping family problems dark is not always possible.

For participants who believed that mental illness was controllable, religious beliefs and practices were seen as important factors. For example, many felt that committing sin could cause mental illness because it was detrimental to one's mental well-being in general.

Participants mentioned a man who had not repented for committing the sin of adultery; they felt that he would be susceptible to mental problems. Because human beings were weak and prone to sinfulness, the willingness to be guided by God could help prevent sins. Other participants said that the work of Satan was shown through anti-social behaviour and psychotic conditions.

Some interviewees related mental illness, including being suicidal, to the original sin committed by Adam and Eve in Eden, which all human beings have inherited and must be punished for. Others believed that mental problems were caused by the Devil, who could assume control of an individual's mind. Mental illness could signify that Satan was testing a person's faith, which in turn helped him or her to perceive the necessity of relying on God. However, some participants questioned the link between Satan and mental disorders. As one pointed out, if mental problems actually were caused by the Devil, psychotropic drugs would not affect them. Even though the participants, and LG Mennonites in general, believed that illness was God-given, mental illness was stigmatized.

Interviewees mentioned extreme examples in which the mentally ill were hidden from public view. In Mexico, a young woman's parents had broken off her relationship with a young man, after which she had a "breakdown" and engaged in out-of-control behaviour, including ripping off her clothes and destroying bedding. As a result, her family confined her in a locked box outside the home. She was not allowed to leave the box, even for meals; instead, food was pushed into it. When concerned neighbours took her in, she behaved in the same fashion. The community speculated that she might be schizophrenic, a condition that commonly manifests during the late teens to early twenties (she was in her late teens). Her frenetic behaviour could support a diagnosis of schizophrenia. We also heard about a young man who exhibited anti-social behaviour after his relationship with a young woman ended. These people may have been negatively judged by the community, but they were still recognized as members of the group, albeit with no distinct role. In some communities, the mentally ill were not seen as capable of contributing to the group and were typically not baptized, because it was believed that they could not understand the significance of the ritual.

Substance Use and Spiritual Health

Participants felt that certain lifestyle choices could contribute to mental illness or lead to it, an opinion that interviewees in the health and illness study also expressed (Kulig et al., 2002). People who chose to drink would continue to stray from God. Some individuals were seen as predisposed to alcoholism, a tendency that was exacerbated by stress. Addiction to alcohol or drugs could affect the brain, which could lead to mental illness. One participant had heard that people who abused drugs burned their brains ("abused drugs dee hauden daut Vestaunt vebrent") and thus were no longer capable of thinking clearly.

Community members believed that the spiritually strong would not drink; as in the study on health and illness, participants in the mental health study stated that people who strayed from God were likely to use and abuse alcohol. In other words, people whose faith was weak drifted away from God and engaged in activities such as drunkenness, a course that simply deepened the estrangement from God. Hence, drinking could interfere with a person's spirituality. Some participants perceived substance abuse as a deliberate flouting of the principles set out by God in the Bible or as grounded in the belief that they need not be obeyed. For these reasons, a few respondents – including a woman whose husband had a drinking problem – saw substance abuse as spiritual illness.

Not all interviewees felt that alcoholism was easily controllable; one woman knew an alcoholic who had tried several times to stop drinking but had not succeeded. Another participant mentioned that ministers could decide whether an individual needed to seek treatment for alcoholism; throughout my years of working with LG Mennonites, I heard many stories of ministers doing this for alcoholics. For instance, when a young man began drinking to excess, the ministers acted to assist him. In such cases, they had determined that alcoholism was a significant problem for the family, had had various unsuccessful talks with the individual, and finally made the extreme decision of ensuring that he received treatment. Some Mennonites in Mexico, Belize, and Bolivia used treatment facilities such as the Centro de Rehabilitación Luz en mi Camino in Cuauhtémoc. A second centre recently opened in Bolivia, which improved access to treatment.

Caring for People with Mental Illness

We heard a number of examples of the difficulty of living with, and caring for, a mentally ill relative. Participants emphasized the importance of keeping oneself well. They said that prayers, reading the Bible, and relying on the strength of God were necessary for getting through each day. Living without stress was also important.

When an LG Mennonite exhibited mental health problems in public, the community could respond in a variety of ways. Participants from Mexico said that mental illness tended not to be understood and that people made fun of afflicted individuals or passed judgment on them or their families. In one case, a man who was mentally unwell could not deal with his farm chores but received no help. Had he been physically ill, community members would normally have assisted him. They could not understand his circumstances, however, and asked, "Wuarom halpt dee sich nich selfst?" (Why does he not help himself?)

Ministers typically provide comfort, support, and guidance to people who are not well and to their family members. During church services, a standard prayer asks God to heal the sick; parishioners who are physically ill are mentioned by name so that the congregation can pray for them, but no mention is made of parishioners who are mentally ill. Overall, our interviewees expressed disappointment in their ministers due to their lack of support for themselves and their mentally unwell relatives. Some who attended conservative churches gave two reasons for the unsatisfactory response. One was that the church leadership understood neither the cause nor the significance of mental illness and had no way of positively relating to afflicted individuals or their family. They simply believed that mental illness was shameful. The other suggestion was that the leadership showed favouritism to certain families; those with a physically unwell relative received support, whereas those with a mentally ill relative did not. In addition, ministers made judgments about the family, especially if alcohol were involved. One woman explained that her father was an alcoholic and that her family had received no support from the church. When her husband became mentally ill, the church continued to ignore their needs in both Mexico and Canada, where they now lived. She believed that this failure to offer help was due to the family history of alcoholism. She mentioned another family in which there was mental illness, but it had received church support. In her opinion, it was helped because it had no record of alcoholism.

The church also failed to help people who experienced the repercussions of alcoholism. One woman told us that her husband drank and physically abused her; her conservative church determined that his behaviour sprang from his lack of mental clarity and that he could not be blamed for it. She was counselled to forgive him for everything he had done to her. Unsurprisingly, she felt that the church had not been supportive in this matter.

A number of interviews shared a common thread: the conservative churches were typically seen as unhelpful, and in fact their treatment of their congregation was perceived as harsh. Their failure to provide support could prompt people to question their faith and sometimes to change churches. One woman explained that her mother had switched to a new church because her original one had not aided her when she had needed assistance in caring for her daughter who had mental health issues. In contrast, my interviews in Durango Colony showed that at least some of the more liberal churches did help people who suffered from mental problems. For example, the ministers counselled those who were struggling and encouraged them to take their medications. Conversely, a visit from a conservative minister implied that someone in the family had acted inappropriately and that a condemnatory message rather than assistance would be the result.

In a few cases, respondents did say that the church had aided the mentally ill. Generally speaking, the most helpful were also the most liberal in nature. In conservative churches, parishioners are not allowed to hold Bible studies and often cannot even read the Bible, which in these churches is usually available only in High German. The liberal churches encourage people to study Scripture, and one participant spoke about how helpful this activity was to her. Another mentioned that, in Mexico, when her daughter developed what was probably bulimia, their minister and his wife visited every week to pray for the girl and to practise the laying on of hands to help her. Church leaders also urged the family to seek medical help, which they acquired from a Mexican physician. Another family in Mexico had experienced a number of suicides. When one of its female members became frightened that she might kill her children, she turned to the church elders for assistance. They agreed to bring Communion to her on a regular basis, which she found helpful in calming her fears.

Our mental health study and our previous studies on other health issues revealed that to LG Mennonites, prayer by unwell individuals or those around them is an important aspect of care. People sometimes resorted to alternative religious treatments. When one of our interviewees learned of a special prayer session that was reputed to heal various disorders, she attended with her husband, who had a mental illness. At the session, they prayed about his problems and attempted to expel the Devil from his body, but his illness did not improve.

Interviewees agreed that community support was necessary in the care of a mentally ill individual, as was being non-judgmental. Engaging in activities with the person, such as going for walks, helped him or her remain active and encouraged thinking about other things. They also mentioned providing meals to diminish the family's workload; although this was commonly done when someone was physically unwell, it was not customary in cases of mental illness.

In Mexico, I met four siblings, all of whom had simple schizophrenia. One brother had agreed to live in the local care facility, leaving his three siblings (two men and a woman) in the family home. They lived in impoverished conditions and exhibited behaviours that the other LG Mennonites in their village perceived as unusual. The church had built them a new house next to the original one, though one brother continued to live in the old home despite its decrepitude. Other kinds of support and care, including food and other resources, were provided to them by several churches and local MCC workers.

Formal Treatment and Care

Participants in our study told us that the parents and siblings of people with mental problems were responsible for the decisions about their care. This differed from the norm for physical illness, where the minister was heavily relied upon for guidance. Families also turned to physicians for aid in making decisions about care.

Treatments and care varied according to location. In both the Cuauhtémoc area and Durango Colony, a Mennonite-managed facility had been established to assist in the care of the mentally ill, including people with schizophrenia. However, not all areas in which LG Mennonites live can boast of such amenities.

Although LG Mennonites commonly do not openly discuss issues relating to mental illness, more liberal-minded Mennonites have a long history of providing services for both the intellectually disabled and the mentally ill. Built in Russia in 1910, Bethania Mental Hospital, the first Mennonite hospital for the mentally ill, operated until 1927 (Huebert, 2011). In North America, the Bethesda Home in Vineland, Ontario, opened in 1937. During the Second World War, Mennonite conscientious objectors worked in Canadian and American mental institutions (Stoesz, 2011), which prompted them to develop facilities elsewhere to ensure that "Christian care" was provided to the mentally ill (Bender, 2011). In Canada, the Eden Mental Health Centre in Winkler, Manitoba, which is run by Eden Health Care Services (EHCS), was established by Manitoba Mennonite churches in 1967 to address the need for more appropriate mental health care (Klassen & Loewen, 2011). This faith-based institution offers both community and in-patient services to LG Mennonites, including addictions counselling. It is still owned by the Mennonite churches of Manitoba but now works in collaboration with Southern Health-Santé Sud in southern Manitoba.[1]

Interviewees described Mexican psychiatric care facilities as less than ideal, whereas many of them talked very positively about the EHCS in southern Manitoba, which they said provided exemplary care not only to clients but also to the family. In fact, some families had left Mexico permanently so that a relative could obtain treatment through the EHCS.

Finally, families and individuals sometimes turned to bone-setters for aid with mental problems. The bone-setter whom I met in Durango Colony talked about assessing the person's feet, where all the nerves accumulate, to discover whether there was tension. This could be relieved by massage, which would help to dispel depression.

Formal care in in-patient or out-patient services included taking medications and seeing a physician and/or psychiatrist on a regular basis. Mentally ill people sometimes had to be hospitalized for treatment.[2] In every case that we heard about, the individual willingly agreed to be admitted.

Participants also talked about prescription medications. Some could name specific types (such as lithium, an anti-psychotic), and some told us that medications could be purchased over the counter in Mexico (as was the case for Haldol, another anti-psychotic). However, most did not know which drug had been prescribed for their relative. We found that over-the-counter medications were not frequently used; when they were, participants were often unable to name the drug or describe the expected result. However, one woman did talk about taking Aspirin to relieve the pain of her depression.

In both Mexico and Canada, it was not uncommon for medications to be distributed and shared among community members.

Respondents who had lived in Mexico and Belize referred to self-proclaimed physicians who prescribed drugs for the mentally ill, though again most could not name these substances or comment on their effectiveness. We were told that using over-the-counter medications or substances from self-proclaimed physicians allowed people with mental issues to conceal their diagnoses from the community.

Unlike individuals with a physical illness, who can count on church and community for care and support, the mentally ill tend to be stigmatized. Caregivers who attempt to help them are commonly left to their own devices. Mental illness is not well understood and is generally perceived as controllable through an effort of will. It is seen as shameful, leaving no choice for individuals but to conceal their symptoms – and, in some cases, for families to hide their relatives away. Our study indicated that prayer and a steadfast belief in God help the mentally ill, while also providing support and strength to caregivers. Some individuals with mental issues use prescription medications, follow the directives of a physician, and agree to hospitalization. Our interviewees felt that if community members could be understanding rather than judgmental, the afflicted would be helped.

CONCLUSION

This book is based on two premises: that religion is an important component in the lives of many people and that cultural competence is essential in supplying them with acceptable and respectful care. The validity of these premises is illustrated by the practices of Low German Mennonites, whose commitment to their faith affects all aspects of their lives, including their beliefs about health and their willingness to use Canada's public health care system.

The book is grounded in a research program that focused on LG Mennonites over a twenty-year period. Through interviews and fieldwork, we discovered how their religious perspectives affected their understanding and experiences of health and illness, women's health, death and dying, and mental health. Our studies consistently reminded us that in the everyday lives of LG Mennonites, religion matters. My hope is that the information shared here will guide those who work directly with LG Mennonites and other Anabaptist groups but also that other caregivers will find it useful in determining the best approach to patients whose faith shapes their response to health care services. I do not suggest that all LG Mennonites believe and express their religion in the same way – individuals may choose to adhere to some principles while discarding others (Fowler, 2009). Health care providers need to be aware of variations between and among groups and individuals, and they must respectfully inquire about beliefs and practices if they wish to plan and implement culturally competent care. Including religion as a variable also recognizes its importance in providing care through a social justice lens (Reimer-Kirkham, 2014).

Several themes emerged during our research. The values and everyday decisions of LG Mennonites are linked to religious beliefs, and these in turn inform their health beliefs and practices. Importantly, the role of suffering in human life was a common theme throughout all our studies, a fact that is fundamental to understanding this group. LG Mennonites see suffering – whether physical, emotional, or spiritual – as a natural part of life. Depending upon their church affiliation, they may see it as a learning opportunity sent by God with the intent of bringing them closer to him, or they may connect it to original sin. People are expected to bear the crosses and burdens that they are given; engaging in daily prayer is therefore an important part of dealing with the difficulties in their lives. In addition, responses to a particular illness or disease are linked with community relationships and perspectives. For example, mental illness is not well understood, and individuals who suffer from it may feel shame and may conceal their disorder to protect themselves and their family from criticism. The use of contraceptives may also be kept secret to avoid the disapproval of community members who espouse certain ideas about regular childbearing.

Suffering and community were just two of the themes that we commonly encountered; others were the use of non-traditional health providers and treatments, the commitment to engage in activities such as prayer and singing to help heal the sick, and the provision of aid to family members to meet their caregiving obligations. Religion helps LG Mennonites understand why illness occurs and how it should be cured. Straying from their principles and hence from God can lead to inappropriate lifestyle choices and associated health problems. Reconnecting with God will resolve this situation and restore health. LG Mennonites will, on their own, combine treatments suggested by traditional and mainstream providers. We learned that one outpatient clinic purposely combines counselling from religious leaders and psychologists, but it was a unique example. Bone-setters diagnose and treat a variety of ailments, including arthritis, and traditional midwives can turn the baby to ensure a normal delivery. Home remedies and over-the-counter medications are also a routine part of self-assigned care plans. If a family member is admitted to hospital, relatives often pray and sing at the bedside, activities that illustrate their commitment to caregiving but also to their religious practices.

Conducting Research among Religiously Diverse Groups

As Canadian society becomes increasingly diverse, it is important to learn about the beliefs and practices of religious groups such as the LG Mennonites. Researchers who study these groups need to develop and apply principles that will ensure the best outcome. Our research principles entailed honesty and transparency in every phase of the project, involving all relevant stakeholders, developing trust with the LG Mennonite participants, and disseminating our findings with consideration of their religious views. These principles are similar to those of participatory action research (Israel, Eng, Schulz, & Parker, 2005), a self-reflective and collaborative approach to public health research. In addition, our efforts extended beyond the consideration of methodology to include reflecting on our personal conduct and that of research assistants during the interviews, at community events, and in the case of the assistants, within their communities. We also established research advisory boards to provide advice and assistance, and we made a point of maintaining participant confidentiality when we reported the highlights of our findings. Finally, we practised self-reflection, assessing our rationale for undertaking the research and the way in which we conducted it. Such self-assessment is essential for research with individuals who are different from oneself. Reflecting on one's own identity and its potential impact on the research process and findings is also important (Nilson, 2017).

Researching religiously diverse groups presents challenges to investigators. For example, they must expect to be questioned about their reasons for undertaking the research, which requires them to reflect upon and explain its moral justification (Liamputtong, 2010). Researchers must sincerely address any concerns raised by respondents. As I interviewed a participant in Durango Colony, he said, "You have asked more questions than I can think of." Interpreting his comment as possibly expressing concern about the research, I explained that I needed to fully understand the topic under investigation, and this helped ease his anxiety. Investigators need to be prepared for the fact that respondents may be subject to social pressure that discourages them from participating. They must also acknowledge that not all members of the group – be they ministers or lay people – will agree with or support the research and that misunderstandings and disagreements may occur about its purpose and the inclusion of group members. Finally, investigators must consider and address power differentials between themselves and the group, as well as within the group, to help foster a positive relationship and ultimately enhance data collection.

Providing Care to Religiously Diverse Groups

Anyone who develops and implements care strategies needs to understand and address the links between religion and health beliefs and practices, whether they relate to health in general or to a specific aspect of it, such as death and dying. Canadians expect that care providers – whether they be registered nurses, social workers, or physicians – will respect their views, religious or otherwise. However, many factors impede this process. Throughout the country, both acute-care and community-based settings are chronically understaffed, and thus the system is overwhelmed by the demands of clients. In such a situation, lack of time often hinders clear communication between provider and client, a problem that is worsened when the latter does not speak fluent English or is uncomfortable in disclosing personal information to a stranger. The lack of translators and interpreters is a common problem;

in southern Alberta, this was addressed by formalizing a full-time position that was mandated to provide translation and to promote understanding of religious beliefs and practices among LG Mennonites.

The issue of gender also has implications for the provision of care to members of diverse religious groups. In the case of LG Mennonite families that attend conservative churches, men typically make the necessary decisions when a relative is ill. Religious leaders, all of whom are male, may also exert significant influence on families that are struggling with ethical questions, such as the use of end-of-life directives or the removal of life support. Furthermore, women's health problems can be overlooked or ignored because their role of providing care for others is seen as more important than caring for themselves. Firmly held convictions or lack of understanding about how the body works can hamper communication about signs and symptoms, and some symptoms and conditions such as depression are seen as controllable by the individual. Women with postpartum depression may be censured as lazy and may thus receive no community or clerical support.

Finally, and perhaps most fundamentally, the LG Mennonite understanding of how the body functions is grounded in religious beliefs and the conviction that differing kinds of illness – physical, mental, and spiritual – are interconnected. Indeed, their belief in spiritual illness as a diagnosis exemplifies their view of an integral relationship between their actions and the power of God. Hence, LG Mennonites feel that individuals who stray from God – and become alcoholics, for example – need spiritual healing just as much as they need physical care. Among those who are preparing for a good death, atoning for sins is crucial; in these circumstances, it is essential that they be permitted to talk with ministers and lay people to exchange forgiveness for transgressions. The constant presence of family and visitors, who commonly pray and sing at the bedside, is a vital part of care for the dying. Privacy at such times is necessary and must be honoured by health care providers.

These examples illustrate the importance of asking questions of the members of any minority religious group – in a manner that displays respect for their beliefs and practices but also does not stereotype them. In addition, it is imperative not to assume that all members of a certain denomination will share the same beliefs. For instance, some conservative LG Mennonite couples feel that women should bear as many children as God wishes, whereas others use contraceptives. However, keeping such decisions confidential is necessary in a community where social pressure often enforces compliance with group norms.

Working collaboratively with LG Mennonites is an important aspect of developing and implementing culturally competent care strategies to address acute or chronic health issues, to foster health promotion, and to prevent illness. One example of an effective partnership is the work of Ruth Babcock (1998); a member of our research advisory group, she conducted her master's research with LG Mennonites in southern Alberta. Using a participatory action research process, she collaborated with community members to develop the HOPE (Help Our People Excel) program, which featured a variety of activities that had a positive impact on health, including health fairs and agricultural safety camps. Babcock's work and its positive outcome are examples of what can be achieved in working with LG Mennonites or any religious group.

Health providers cannot generate effective cultural competence principles in isolation. Discussions of diversity and its implications for health care must become central to all educational programs for health professionals. Some commentators have urged that cultural competency content be added to the nursing curriculum (Mareno & Hart, 2014), but this would be just the first step. Health regions must offer continuing education programs to teach caregivers about the diverse religious groups in their area, concentrating on how to provide appropriate care. To accomplish this, education and professional development should focus on nurturing a collaborative process between providers and clients, leading to optimum levels of satisfaction for individuals, families, religious leaders, and all stakeholders in the health care system.

Policy Implications

Canada's official multiculturalism policy was developed to address the changing nature of our society. Focusing primarily on ethnicity and race, it was intended to help integrate members of diverse groups into all aspects of Canadian life. Although policy makers originally believed that the Multiculturalism Act would apply to religious convictions as well, some policy experts feel that it has not sufficiently done so (Kunz, 2009; Fadden & Townsend, 2009), and there have been calls to address religious diversity more formally in Canada. In addition, religious diversity tends to be associated with immigrants and refugees rather than with people who have lived in Canada for some time but whose faith is not widely understood. The LG Mennonites are a good example of the latter: although they have resided in this country since the late nineteenth century, most Canadians are unfamiliar with their beliefs and know virtually nothing about their daily lives.

According to policy experts, when issues arise that are related to religious diversity, the appropriate solution may lie at the micro, meso, or macro level (Kunz, 2009). At the micro level, private organizations and individuals apply mutually agreed upon strategies to resolve problems. Public policy interventions typically do not occur at this level, and most differences are privately resolved between those who are immediately affected. One example of a micro strategy occurred in a long-term-care facility where most residents were Mennonites. Due to a decrease in staff, its routines had to be adjusted, with the result that residents could now be bathed on Sundays. This day was normally reserved for family visits and prayer, so the members of the board – which included local Mennonite ministers from a range of churches – had to be provided with information to help them understand the change. After the explanation was given, they agreed that the new routine was both necessary and acceptable.

At the meso level, public policies, programs, and services from all levels of government are tailored to adhere to the core values of Canada's Constitution (Kunz, 2009). It is at this level that the health care system is situated; policies in institutions such as hospitals or in community settings such as public health offices must be adapted to address religious diversity. A simple example here would be the development of a policy to accommodate multiple visitors in a hospital room, while also respecting the privacy and other needs of visitors who practise activities such as prayer and the laying on of hands. Health managers may assert that such policies are already in place, but our research revealed that some LG Mennonites were made to feel uncomfortable when they prayed and sang at the bedside. Ongoing policy reviews and evaluations, comparing what is written with what actually occurs, are helpful in assessing and improving the situation.

Finally, at the macro level, all citizens must be treated with respect regardless of their background – which is not the same as receiving privileges that the core values of society do not support. Such measures can be implemented only through national policies (Kunz, 2009). Like any group, the LG Mennonites whom this book discusses are constantly subject to change. In years to come, they may discard some of the beliefs and practices that are presented here. Nonetheless, they are an excellent case example of the importance of acknowledging and understanding religious diversity in our society and of using cultural competence to provide respectful care that is grounded in a collaborative process. To achieve this, care providers need both appropriate education and supportive health care organizations. However, a policy environment that respects religious diversity is equally essential because it provides direction for health care organizations in formulating their mission and goals. Canada has always been a diverse country; it is therefore important for all of us to understand issues relating to diversity and to invest time and effort in more fully understanding those around us. If we work hard and are fortunate, our society will become increasingly inclusive, and all of us will enjoy equity in every area of life.

NOTES

Introduction

1 In discussing LG Mennonites, I use the word "diverse" to avoid invoking the power differentials that are inherent in words such as "vulnerable" and "marginalized."

2 The request for a cultural assessment originally came from Barons-Eureka-Warner Health Unit, which was later amalgamated with other units, becoming collectively known as the Chinook Regional Health Authority. Various other mergers have since taken place, and now the entire province is served by just one body: Alberta Health Services.

3 For health and illness, see Hall & Kulig (2004); Hall, Kulig, Campbell, Wall, & Babcock (2005); Kulig et al. (2002); and Kulig & Hall (2004). For women's health and sexuality, see Kulig, Hall, Babcock, Campbell, & Wall (2004), Kulig, Babcock, Wall, & Hill (2006, 2009) and Kulig, Wall, Hill, & Babcock (2008). For death and dying, see Kulig & Fan (2013a, 2013b, 2013c); and Fan & Kulig (2014). For mental health, see Kulig & Fan (2016a, 2016b). All these studies included a research advisory group whose members represented the respective health and social services region(s) in the province(s) where the projects were conducted, as well as from the Mennonite Central Committee. The local research assistants whom we hired were Mennonites who spoke fluent Plautdietsch.

4 Undertaking research with this group involves many challenges, particularly among the more conservative LG Mennonites. These include language barriers, the need to establish and maintain trust, the rejection of technology by some LG Mennonites, their concerns about disclosing sensitive information to others, and their emphasis on living separately from mainstream society (Hall & Kulig, 2004).

Mennonite scholarship has focused largely on immigration history and religious perspectives or the work of Mennonite missionaries. Research among Mennonites has been either group-specific (e.g., Bolivian Mennonites) or limited to particular topics, such as cultural identity (Warkentin, 2010), agricultural practices (Higdon, 1997), or community fragmentation (Kok & Roessingh, 2013). Fehr Keller (2006) discusses preservation and transmission of culture among LG Mennonites in southern Manitoba. Mennonite researchers have not directly focused their research on health issues relating to LG Mennonites in Canada or elsewhere. However, a non-Mennonite, Reinschmidt (2001), concentrated on the Cuauhtémoc area of Mexico and examined the lives of LG Mennonite women in relation to health and illness. Two other non-Mennonites conducted research among this population: Hedges (1996) examined language and identity among Old Colony Mennonites in Cuauhtémoc, a topic that can relate to LG Mennonites' access to health services and care; and Cañás Bottos (2008) studied community life and change among LG Mennonites in Argentina and Bolivia and, in so doing, identified impacts on their well-being.

5 Once the Mennonite liaison worker was hired, she also joined the advisory group. In the women's health study, this group was limited to female members, but for the other studies it included both women and men.

6 Generally speaking, the RAs had Mennonite backgrounds. In one exceptional case, when the local RA was unable to do so, LingLing Fan (not a Mennonite) handled the interviewing.

7 The decision not to record our interviews was based on advice from the late Dr. Leonard Sawatzky, who followed the same routine and successfully worked with Mennonites in Mexico (Sawatzky, 1971). Refraining from tape recording enhanced our relationship with participants and helped them to speak freely.

8 The data analysis process is described in more detail in Hall & Kulig (2004), Kulig & Fan (2013b), and Kulig, Wall, Hill, Babcock (2008).

9 LingLing (HaiYan) Fan was project coordinator for the death and dying (2009–14) and mental health studies (2012–16) (for the former, see Kulig & Fan, 2013a, 2013b, 2013c; Fan & Kulig, 2014; for the latter, see Kulig & Fan, 2016a, 2016b). Her master's thesis, which dealt with death and dying (Fan, 2011), focused on ideas about palliative care and was grounded in fieldwork that she undertook in Cuauhtémoc, southern Alberta, and Manitoba.

Chapter 1: A Brief History of the Low German Mennonites

1 *Strasse* is the German word for "street," and *dorf* means "village."

2 Old Colony Mennonites should not be confused with Old Order Mennonites, whose practices include the use of horses and buggies for transportation.

3 Official statistics for the LG Mennonite population in Canada and elsewhere are not available. Unless otherwise indicated, the figures presented here are estimates provided by former and current employees of Mennonite Central Committee Canada.

4 The decision to excommunicate or ban an individual lies with the church leadership, which may bar a person from attending church and community services. This penalty can be rescinded if the individual repents and refrains from the inappropriate behaviour. However, if the behaviour persists, the leadership will take further punitive measures.

Chapter 2: Health and Illness

1 The use of the term "lady doctor" was common among participants to identify self-taught health care providers. The trained physicians the participants consulted in Mexico were generally male, while alternative health providers, particularly for women's health, were generally female.

Chapter 5: Mental Health

1 In this instance, "community" refers to their neighbours and personal networks, not their church connections.

2 Under the terms of the Mental Health Act, individuals who become a danger to themselves or others must be taken into psychiatric care. This normally includes a police escort to the facility to ensure that no one is harmed along the way.

REFERENCES

Alizadeh, S., & Chavan, M. (2016). Cultural competence dimensions and outcomes: A systematic review of the literature. *Health and Social Care in the Community, 24*, e117–30.

Babcock, R. (1998). *Participatory action research with the German speaking Mennonites* (Unpublished master's thesis). University of Lethbridge, AB.

Bender, T. (2011). The Mennonite mental health movement and the wider society in the United States, 1942–1965. *Journal of Mennonite Studies, 29*, 45–60.

Blanchet Garneau, A. (2013). *Proposition théorique constructiviste du développement de la compétence culturelle infirmière* [Constructivist theoretical proposition for the development of cultural competence in nursing] (Unpublished doctoral dissertation). Université de Montréal, QC.

Blanchet Garneau, A. (2016). Critical reflection in cultural competence development: A framework for undergraduate nursing eduation. *Journal of Nursing Education, 55*, 125–32.

Blanchet Garneau, A., & Pepin, J. (2015). Cultural competence: A constructivist definition. *Journal of Transcultural Nursing, 26*, 9–15.

Brascoupe, S., & Waters, C. (2009). Exploring the applicability of the concept of cultural safety to Aboriginal health and community wellness. *Journal of Aboriginal Health, 5*, 6–41.

Braun, V., & Clarke, V. (2006). Using thematic analysis in psychology. *Qualitative Research in Psychology, 3*, 77–101.

Brenneman, G. (1979). Abortion: Review of Mennonite literature, 1970–1977. *Mennonite Quarterly Review, 53*, 160–72.

Burrill, E. (1998). *Health conception, family health work and health promoting lifestyle practices in Latin American Mennonite families* (Unpublished master's thesis). University of Western Ontario, London, ON.

Campinha-Bacote, J. (2002). The process of cultural competence in the delivery of healthcare services: A model of care. *Journal of Transcultural Nursing, 13*, 181–84.

Cañás Bottos, L. (2008). *Old Colony Mennonites in Argentina and Bolivia: Nation making, religious conflict and imagination of the future.* Boston: Brill Academic.

Castro, P. (2004). The 'return' of the Mennonites from the Cuauhtémoc region to Canada: A perspective from Mexico. *Journal of Mennonite Studies, 22*, 25–38.

Cox, C. (2008). *Mennonite Plautdietsch – Language and history* [PowerPoint presentation slides]. Retrieved from http://mhss.sk.ca/Gen/cox/index.shtml.

De, D., & Richardson, J. (2008). Cultural safety: An introduction. *Paediatric Nursing, 20*, 39–43.

Dreachslin, J., Gilbert, M.J., & Malone, B. (2013). *Diversity and cultural competence in health care: A systems approach.* San Francisco: Jossey-Bass.

Driedger, L. (2000). *Mennonites in the global village.* Toronto: University of Toronto Press.

Dyck, C.J. (1967). *An introduction to Mennonite history: A popular history of the Anabaptists and Mennonites.* Waterloo, ON: Herald Press.

Enns, K. (2009). Old Colony Mennonites of Mexico: A separate people. *California Mennonite Historical Society Bulletin, 50*, 1–6. Retrieved from https://fpuscholarworks.fresno.edu/bitstream/handle/11418/90/CMHS050-1.pdf.

Epp, M. (1987). Women in Canadian Mennonite history: Uncovering the 'underside.' *Journal of Mennonite Studies, 5*, 90–107.

Erlen, J. (1998). Culture, ethics, and respect: The bottom line is understanding. *Orthopaedic Nursing, 17*, 79–82.

Fadden, R., & Townsend, T. (2009). Dealing with religious diversity: Opportunities and challenges. *Horizons, 10*(2), 4–5. Retrieved from http://www.horizons.gc.ca/sites/default/files/Publication-alt-format/2009-0008-eng.pdf.

Fan, H. (2011). *Medical encounters in "closed religious communities": Palliative care for Low German-speaking Mennonite people* (Unpublished master's thesis). University of Lethbridge, AB.

Fan, H., & Kulig, J. (2014). Health care in rural settings: Palliative care for the Low German Mennonites. *Journal of Rural Community Development, 9*, 246–58.

Fast, K., & Epp Buller, R. (2013). Introduction. In R. Epp Buller & K. Fast (Eds.), *Mothering Mennonite* (pp. 1–19). Bradford, ON: Demeter Press.

Fehr Keller, T. (2006). *The preservation and transmission of culture and religion among Dietsche (Low German) Mennonite returnees to southern Manitoba* (Unpublished master's thesis). University of Manitoba, Winnipeg.

Felt, J., Ridley, J., Allen, G., & Redekop, C. (1990). High fertility of Old Colony Mennonites in Mexico. *Human Biology, 62*, 689–700.

Fowler, M. (2009). Religion, bioethics and nursing practice. *Nursing Ethics, 16*, 393–405.

Friesen, J. (2011). Reinlander Mennoniten Gemeinde. In D.F. Plett (Ed.), *Old Colony Mennonites in Canada: 1875 to 2000* (pp. 3–19). Winnipeg: D.F. Plett Historical Research Foundation.

Gingrich, L. (2013). Preserving cultural heritage in the context of migratory livelihoods. *International Migration, 52*, 1–20.

Gingrich, L., & Loewen, J.B. (2013). Belize. In *Global Anabaptist Mennonite encyclopedia online.* Retrieved from http://gameo.org/index.php?title=Belize.

Guenther, B. (2004). A road less traveled: The evangelical path of Kanadier Mennonites who returned to Canada. *Journal of Mennonite Studies, 22*, 143–66.

Hall, B., & Kulig, J. (2004). Kanadier Mennonites: A case study examining research challenges among religious groups. *Qualitative Health Research, 14*(3), 359–68.

Hall, B., Kulig, J., Campbell, R., Wall, M., & Babcock, R. (2005). Social work and Kanadier Mennonites: Challenges and rewards. *Journal of Religion and Spirituality in Social Work: Social Thought, 24*, 91–104.

Hedges, K.L. (1996). *'Plautdietsch' and 'Huuchdietsch' in Chihuahua: Language, literacy, and identity among the Old Colony Mennonites in northern Mexico* (Doctoral dissertation). Retrieved from UMI Dissertation Services.

Hickman, J. (2006). *Faith community nursing.* Philadelphia: Lippincott Williams & Wilkins.

Higdon, F. (1997). *Farm diversification and specialization: The adaptation of Mennonite households in Spanish Lookout, Belize farm households* (Doctoral dissertation). Retrieved from UMI Dissertation Services.

Huebert, H. (2011). The Bethania Mental Hospital of Russia, 1910–1927. *Journal of Mennonite Studies, 29*, 215–19.

Hurst, B. (2003). *The articulation of Mennonite beliefs about sexuality, 1890–1930* (Doctoral dissertation). Retrieved from Abstracts International, UMI No. 3087208.

Israel, B.A., Eng, E., Schulz, A.J., & Parker, E.A. (2005). *Methods in community-based participatory research for health.* San Francisco: Jossey-Bass.

Janzen, J. (2010). Hemispheric approach [Notes]. Mennonite Central Committee Networking Meeting, Steinreich Bible School, Cuauhtémoc, Mexico.

Janzen, W. (2004). Welcoming the returning 'Kanadier' Mennonites from Mexico. *Journal of Mennonite Studies, 22*, 11–24.

Janzen, W. (2007). *Why did they leave Canada? The Mennonite migration to Mexico and Paraguay in the 1920s.* Ottawa: Mennonite Central Committee Canada.

Johnston, B., Kulig, J., Campbell, R., Turcato, G., Babcock R., & Scovill, S. (1997, May). *Kanadier (Mexican) Mennonites: Meeting the nutritional needs of special populations.* Poster presented at Working in Public Health, Alberta Public Health Association Annual Conference, Calgary.

Kezios, L.K., Liu, Z., Cirillo, P.M., Cohn, B.A., Kalantzi, O. I., Wang, Y., Petreas, M.X., Park, J.-S., & Factor-Litvak, P. (2013). Dichlorodiphenyltrichloroethane (DDT), DDT metabolites and pregnancy outcomes. *Reproductive Toxicology, 35,* 156–64. Retrieved from http://www.sciencedirect.com/science/article/pii/S0890623812003164.

Klassen, G., & Loewen, C. (2011). Before Eden: The Evangelical Mennonite Conference and the founding of a mental health facility. *Journal of Mennonite Studies, 29,* 105–19.

Kok, A., & Roessingh, C. (2013). Where 'God sleeps at night': Integration, differentiation and fragmentation in a Mennonite colony. *Journal of Mennonite Studies, 31,* 167–82.

Krahn, C., & Sawatzky, H.L. (1990). Old Colony Mennonites. In *Global Anabaptist Mennonite encyclopedia online.* Retrieved from http://gameo.org/index.php?title=Old_Colony_Mennonites.

Kulig, J. (1995). *Community assessment of the Kanadier (Mexican) Mennonites.* Lethbridge, AB: Regional Centre for Health Promotion and Community Studies, University of Lethbridge. Retrieved from https://www.uleth.ca/dspace/bitstream/handle/10133/785/Community_Assessment_of_the_Kanadier_(Mexican)_Mennonites.pdf.

Kulig, J., Babcock, R., Wall, M., & Hill, S. (2006). *Growing up as a woman: The health perspectives of Low-German-speaking Mennonite women.* Lethbridge, AB: University of Lethbridge.

Kulig, J., Babcock, R., Wall, M., & Hill, S. (2009). Being a woman: Perspectives of Low German-speaking Mennonite women. *Health Care for Women International, 30,* 324–38.

Kulig, J., & Fan, H. (2011). Suffering: Is the concept significant among Low German-speaking Mennonites? *Journal of Mennonite Studies, 29,* 153–65.

Kulig, J., & Fan, H. (2013a). *Best practices for diverse populations: End-of-life care among the Low German-speaking Mennonites.* Lethbridge, AB: University of Lethbridge.

Kulig, J., & Fan, H. (2013b). *Death and dying beliefs and practices among Low German-speaking Mennonites: Application to practice.* Lethbridge, AB: University of Lethbridge.

Kulig, J., & Fan, H. (2013c). Understanding death and dying among the Low German-speaking Mennonites: Perspectives from a closed religious group. *Journal of Hospice and Palliative Nursing Care, 15,* 52–59.

Kulig, J., & Fan, H. (2016a). *Cultural guidelines to support mental health among the Low German Mennonites.* Lethbridge, AB: University of Lethbridge. Retrieved from https://www.uleth.ca/dspace/bitstream/handle/10133/4496/Kulig%20Cultural%20Guidelines%20to%20Support%20Mental%20Health....pdf.

Kulig, J., & Fan, H. (2016b). *Mental health beliefs and practices among Low German Mennonites: Application to practice.* Lethbridge, AB: University of Lethbridge. Retrieved from https://www.uleth.ca/dspace/bitstream/handle/10133/4510/Kulig%20ULeth_mental_health_final_LR.pdf.

Kulig, J., & Hall, B. (2004). Health and illness beliefs among southern Alberta Kanadier Mennonites. *Journal of Mennonite Studies, 22,* 185–204.

Kulig, J., Hall, B., Babcock, R., Campbell, R., & Wall, M. (2004). Childbearing knowledge, beliefs and practices among Kanadier Mennonite women. *Canadian Nurse, 100,* 34–37.

Kulig, J., Hall, B., Wall, M., Janzen, W., Campbell, R., & Babcock, R. (2002). *Kanadier Mennonites: Gaining an understanding of their health and illness beliefs.* Lethbridge, AB: University of Lethbridge.

Kulig, J., & McCaslin, C. (1998). Mexican Mennonites: A group in transition. *Canadian Nurse, 94,* 34–39.

Kulig, J., Wall, M., Hill, S., & Babcock, R. (2008). Childbearing beliefs among Low-German-speaking Mennonite women. *International Nursing Review, 55,* 420–26.

Kunz, J. (2009). Religious diversity in a multicultural Canada: Quo vadis? *Horizons, 10*(2), 6–13. Retrieved from http://www.horizons.gc.ca/sites/default/files/Publication-alt-format/2009-0008-eng.pdf.

Lehman, D., Fenza, P., & Hollinger-Smith, L. (2012). *Diversity and cultural competency in health care settings.* Evanston, IL: Mather LifeWays.

Liamputtong, P. (2010). *Performing qualitative cross-cultural research.* New York: Cambridge University Press.

Liamputtong, P. (2013). *Qualitative research methods* (4th ed.). Melbourne: Oxford University Press.

Loewen, R. (1993). *Family, church and market: A Mennonite community in the old and new worlds, 1850–1930.* Toronto: University of Toronto Press.

Loewen, R. (2001). *Hidden worlds.* Winnipeg: University of Manitoba Press.

Loewen, R. (2013). *Village among nations: "Canadian" Mennonites in a transnational world, 1916–2006.* Toronto: University of Toronto Press.

Mareno, N., & Hart, P. (2014). Cultural competency among nurses with undergraduate and graduate degrees: Implications for nursing education. *Nursing Education Perspectives, 35,* 83–88.

Narayanasamy, A., & White, E. (2005). A review of transcultural nursing. *Nurse Education Today, 25,* 102–11.

Newman Giger, J. (2012). *Transcultural nursing: Assessment and intervention.* Toronto: Elsevier.

Nilson, C. (2017). A journey toward cultural competence: The role of researcher reflexivity in Indigenous research. *Journal of Transcultural Nursing, 28,* 119–27.

Parisa, B., Reza, N., Afsaneh, R., & Sarieh, P. (2016). Cultural safety: An evolutionary concept analysis. *Holistic Nursing Practice, 30,* 33–38.

Pauls, K. (2004). Northfield Settlement, Nova Scotia: A new direction for immigrants from Belize. *Journal of Mennonite Studies, 22*, 167–84.

Penner, C.J. (1999). *Mennonite silences and feminist voices: Peace theology and violence against women* (Unpublished doctoral dissertation). Toronto School of Theology.

Pesut, B., Fowler, M., Taylor, E., Reimer-Kirkham, S., & Sawatzky, R. (2008). Conceptualising spirituality and religion for healthcare. *Journal of Clinical Nursing, 17*, 2803–10.

Plasil, T. (2009). Processes of change in Shipyard. In C. Roessingh & T. Plasil (Eds.), *Between horse and buggy and four-wheel drive: Change and diversity among Mennonite settlements in Belize, Central America* (pp. 117–47). Amsterdam: VU University Press.

Plasil, T., & Roessingh, C. (2009). The Mennonite road to Belize. In C. Roessingh & T. Plasil (Eds.), *Between horse and buggy and four-wheel drive: Change and diversity among Mennonite settlements in Belize, Central America* (pp. 43–72). Amsterdam: VU University Press.

Polaschek, N.R. (1998). Cultural safety: A new concept in nursing people of different ethnicities. *Journal of Advanced Nursing, 27*, 452–57.

Quadros, D. (2009). *Experiences of Mennonite immigrant women accessing and receiving services in the mental health care system in Essex County* (Unpublished master's thesis). University of Windsor, London, ON.

Quiring, D. (1997). *Mennonite colony life: Under siege in Mexico* (Unpublished master's thesis). University of Saskatchewan, Saskatoon.

Reimer-Kirkham, S. (2014). Nursing research on religion and spirituality through a social justice lens. *Advances in Nursing Science, 37*, 249–57.

Reinschmidt, K.M. (2001). *Old Colony and General Conference Mennonites in Chihuahua, Mexico: History, representations and women's everyday lives in health and illness* (Doctoral dissertation). Retrieved from UMI Dissertation Services.

Rempel, H. (1984). *Kjenn Jie Noch Plautdietsch? A Mennonite Low German dictionary.* Winnipeg: Mennonite Literary Society.

Sawatzky, H.L. (1971). *They sought a country: Mennonite colonization in Mexico.* Berkeley: University of California Press.

Sawatzky, R.M. (2005). *The control of social space in Mennonite housebarns of Manitoba, 1874–1940* (Unpublished doctoral dissertation). Simon Fraser University, Burnaby, BC.

Shen, Z. (2015). Cultural competence models and cultural competence assessment instruments in nursing: A literature review. *Journal of Transcultural Nursing, 26*, 308–21.

Smith, H. (1981). *The story of the Mennonites.* Berne, IN: Mennonite Book Concern.

Stoesz, C. (2011). 'Are you prepared to work in a mental hospital?' Canadian conscientious objectors' service during the Second World War. *Journal of Mennonite Studies*, 29, 61–73.

Urry, J. (2006). *Mennonites, politics and peoplehood: Europe, Canada, 1525–1980*. Winnipeg: University of Manitoba Press.

Visser, P. (2009). Preface. In C. Roessingh & T. Plasil (Eds.), *Between horse and buggy and four-wheel drive: Change and diversity among Mennonite settlements in Belize, Central America* (pp. 7–9). Amsterdam: VU University Press.

Warkentin, K. (2010). *'So Ha' Wie Daut Emma Jedohne' (That is how we have always done it): The collective memory and cultural identity of the Old Colony Mennonites in Bolivia* (Unpublished master's thesis). University of Manitoba, Winnipeg.

Wenger, M. (2000). *Anointing the sick with oil in the Mennonite Church: An exercise in practical theology* (Unpublished doctoral dissertation). Faculty of Union Theological Seminary and Presbyterian School of Christian Education, Richmond, VA.

Wepa, D. (2003). An exploration of the experiences of cultural safety educators in New Zealand: An action research approach. *Journal of Transcultural Nursing*, 14, 339–48.

Wiebe Krahn, H. (2012). *Poor but clean: The story of my life from Mexico through Canada and Central America to Australia*. Detention River, Tasmania: Rocky Cape Christian Community.

Wood, P., & Schwass, M. (1993). Cultural safety: A framework for changing attitudes. *Nursing Praxis in New Zealand*, 8, 4–15.

Zacharias, E. (2009). *Ons leeschtet Wieedabuak: Low German dictionary*. Winnipeg: Commonword Bookstore.

INDEX

abortion, 58–59, 67–69. *See also* miscarriage
afterlife beliefs, 87
alcohol and alcoholism: beliefs about, 47, 101; beliefs about fetal impact, 70, 71; excommunication for, 88; prevalence and impacts, 16, 42; support and treatment, 16, 44–45, 51, 101–2, 103
amputated body parts, burial of, 89
Anabaptist movement, 21
angels, 83
anointing, with water or oil, 83
arthritis, 43, 49, 51

Babcock, Ruth, 114
baby blues, 73, 98. *See also* postpartum depression
Belize: abortion practices, 68; access to medication and health services, 50, 52, 60–61; author's research in, 12–13; DDT use for household cleaning, 41; migration to, 26; population of Low German Mennonites, 31; preparation of bodies for burial, 86; substance abuse treatment, 102
Bethania Mental Hospital (Russia), 105
Bethesda Home (Vineland, ON), 105
Bible: evangelical movement on, 26; interpretation and study of, 33, 55, 104; Menno Simons on, 21; role in daily life, 9, 52; role in spiritual health, 96
bipolar disorder, 98
birth control, 65–67, 110, 114
Bolivia, 26, 31, 102
bone-setters, 13, 48, 51–52, 61, 106, 111
brain death, 85
breastfeeding, 73–74
Brenneman, George, 58–59
burial. *See* funerals and burial
burns, 43, 51
Burrill, Elizabeth, 41, 49

Cañás Bottos, Lorenzo, 45, 117*n*4
caregiving: of disabled individuals, 53–54; discussing issues with family members, 54; of dying individuals, 81; elder care, 53; liaison workers, 52–53; responsibility for, 52, 54, 61–62
Chihuahua. *See* Mexico

childbirth, 72–73
children: attendance at funerals, 86–87; burial of, 90; education, 24, 34, 36; genetic disorders, 53, 70; *Kopp Krankheit*, 43, 51; nutritional issues, 42; support for orphans, 91. *See also* pregnancy and childbirth
Chinook Regional Health Authority, 10, 117*n*2
cleanliness, 41
clergy. *See* ministers
colds, 49
collaborative approaches, 114
community events, 14–15
contraceptives. *See* birth control
cremation, 86
Cuauhtémoc. *See* Mexico
cultural awareness, 5
cultural beliefs and practices, 4
cultural competence: approach to, 4–5, 109; Cultural Competence Development Model, 6–8; definition, 5–6, 6–7; education and professional development for, 114; role in health care, 6; for working with Low German Mennonites, 17–19, 109–10
cultural sensitivity, 5

DDT, 41
death and dying: afterlife beliefs, 87; anointing with water or oil, 83; beliefs about, 80; brain death, 85; caregiving for, 81; end-of-life directives, 84; euthanasia, 85; interview participants, 79; introduction and conclusions, 79, 91; laying on of hands, 83; life support, 84–85; organ donation, 85; palliative care, 83–84; preparations for death, 82–83, 113; suffering during, 48, 83; support for orphans, widows, and widowers, 90–91; unexpected death, 80–81. *See also* funerals and burial
dental health, 40
depression, 44, 74, 94, 98. *See also* postpartum depression
diabetes, type 1, 53
diarrhea, 49
Dietsche speakers, use of term, 30
disabilities, 45, 53–54
diverse, use of term, 117*n*1
domestic violence, 42, 75–76
drugs. *See* substance abuse
Durango. *See* Mexico

eating disorders, 98
eczema, 50
Eden Health Care Services (EHCS), 105–6
Eden Mental Health Centre (Winkler, MB), 105
education, 24, 34, 36
elder care, 53
end-of-life directives, 84
Epp, Marlene, 56, 59
Epp Buller, Rachel, 36
euthanasia, 85
Evangelical Mennonite Church (Kleine Gemeinde), 32–33, 34
Evangelical Mennonite Mission Church, 32–33, 36
evangelical movement, 26–27
excommunication, 28, 35, 68, 88, 119*n*4

faith-based community, 31
Fan, HaiYan (LingLing), 13, 90, 118*n*6, 118*n*9
Fast, Kerry, 36
Fehr Keller, T., 117*n*4
folk remedies, 51
food, 41–42
funerals and burial: of amputated body parts, 89; attendance of children, 86–87; burial practices,

86; cremation, 86; of excommunicants, 88; funeral service, 87; of infants and children, 90; lack of support during, 87; preparation of body, 86; of suicides, 88–89; as teaching opportunities, 89. *See also* death and dying

gender roles and issues, 58, 113
genetic disorders, 53, 70
gossip, 94–95, 99

hands, laying on of, 83
headscarf, 36, 58
health and illness: beliefs about, 40–41, 60; interview participants, 39–40; introduction and conclusions, 39–40, 54; suffering, 45–48, 75, 83, 110; types of illness, 42–45; unhealthy practices, 42; values associated with health, 41–42. *See also* caregiving; death and dying; mental health and illness; pregnancy and childbirth; treatment; women's health
Health Options Scale, 41
Health-Promoting Lifestyle Profile II, 41
Hedges, K.L., 117*n*4
honour, family, 63
HOPE (Help Our People Excel) program, 114
Hurst, Brenda, 58
hygiene, 41
hysterectomy, 74

illness. *See* health and illness

Janzen, John, 31

Kanadiers, use of term, 30
Kleine Gemeinde (Evangelical Mennonite Church), 32–33, 34
Kopp Krankheit, 43, 51

La Crete (AB), 13
lady doctor, 51, 61, 64, 66, 72, 119*n*1 (chap. 2)
language usage, 8–9
laying on of hands, 83
liaison workers, 10, 52–53, 61, 72, 112–13, 118*n*5
life support, 84–85
Loewen, Royden, 29, 56
Low German, use of term, 30
Low German Mennonites: cultural competence for working with, 17–19, 109–10; denominations and religious variation, 32–33; education, 24, 34, 36; excommunication, 35; as faith-based community, 31–32; health care interactions, 37; language usage, 8–9; introduction, 8–9; population estimates, 31, 119*n*3; religious beliefs, 9, 17, 21, 26–27, 28, 33–34; religious beliefs and health care, 18–19, 109–11; scholarship on, 117*n*4; separation from world, 32, 34–35; social relationships, 11; technology usage, 9, 36–37; terminology for, 30–31; women's clothing and appearance, 35–36
Low German Mennonites, author's interactions and research: challenges faced, 117*n*4; changes among Low German Mennonites and, 16–17; concerns by Low German Mennonites, 14–16; justification and affirmation of research, 11–12; overview, 9–11; research process and fieldwork, 12–14, 111, 117*n*3, 118*nn*5–7
Low German Mennonites, history: Anabaptist roots, 21; changes among Canadian Mennonites,

26–27; changes among Latin American Mennonites, 29; external threats in Canada, 24–25; introduction and conclusions, 21, 37; Manitoba settlements, 23; migration to North America, 22–23; migrations back to Canada, 27–28; migrations to Latin America, 25–26; migrations within Canada, 24; religious differences and migration, 28; in Russia, 22

marriage, 58, 90
medication, 47, 50, 52, 95–96, 106–7. *See also* treatment
Mennonite Central Committee (MCC), 12, 61
Mennonites, 21. *See also* Low German Mennonites
menstruation, 64–65
Mental Health Act, 119*n*2 (chap. 5)
mental health and illness: beliefs about causes and ability to cope, 44, 94, 95, 96–98, 110; depression, 44, 74, 94, 98; formal treatment and care, 105–7; interview participants, 93–94; introduction and conclusions, 93–94, 107; Mental Health Act, 119*n*2 (chap. 5); *narvenkrankheit*, 44, 94; perception of mentally ill, 100–1; postpartum depression, 18, 73, 98–99, 113; scholarship on, 94–96; spiritual health and, 96, 99–100; stigmatization and attempts to hide illness, 94–95, 99, 100; substance abuse, 101–2; support from church and community, 74, 95–96, 102–5; value of positive, 42
Mexican Mennonites, use of term, 30
Mexico: access to medication and health services, 50, 52, 60–61; author's research in, 13; care for disabled, 53–54; common physical illnesses, 43; diet, 42; education, 36; migration to and from, 25, 26, 27–28, 29; population of Low German Mennonites, 31; preparation of bodies for burial, 86; substance abuse treatment, 102; support for orphans, 90–91; treatment in, 48–52
ministers: biblical interpretation role, 33, 55; concerns about author's research, 14; dying individuals and, 82, 85; on life support, 85; responses to alcoholism, 44, 101–2, 103; role in health care, 18–19; sermons at funerals, 89
miscarriage, 59, 70, 74–75. *See also* abortion
motherhood, 57
multiculturalism, 3, 115
Muslim immigrants and refugees, 3

***n**arvenkrankheit*, 44, 94. *See also* depression
nerve pills, 73
Northfield Settlement (NS), 26
nutrition, 41–42

oil, anointing with, 83
Old Colony Mennonite Church (Rheinlander Church), 32
Old Colony Mennonites: on excommunication, 35; geography and religious variation, 33; migration by, 25; on separation from world, 34; technology usage, 36; use of term, 23, 30, 119*n*2 (chap. 1)
Old Order Mennonites, 119*n*2 (chap. 1)
old-age homes, 53
Ordnung, 32, 34
organ donation, 85
orphans, 91

palliative care, 83–84
Paraguay, 25–26, 29
participatory action research, 111
physical illness, 43
Plautdietsch, 8
policy, and religious diversity, 115–16
population, Low German Mennonite, 31, 119*n*3
postpartum depression, 18, 73, 98–99, 113
pregnancy and childbirth: abortion, 58–59, 67–69; birth control, 65–67, 110, 114; breastfeeding, 73–74; childbirth, 72–73; miscarriage, 59, 70, 74–75; postpartum depression, 18, 73, 98–99, 113; postpartum support, 73–74; prenatal care and beliefs, 69–72; reproduction beliefs, 65; "turning the baby," 71

Quadros, Diane, 95
Quiring, David, 34, 35

Reinschmidt, Kerstin: on death and dying, 80; on funerals, 87; on health and illness definitions, 40; on mental health, 94; on physical illness, 43; scholarship by, 59–60, 117*n*4; on suffering, 45; on treatments, 48, 50
religiously diverse groups: approach to, 3–4, 109; common perceptions of, 3, 115; vs cultural diversity, 4; need for cultural competence for addressing, 4–5; policy implications, 115–16; providing care to, 112–14; research among, 111–12. *See also* cultural competence
reproduction, 65
Rheinlander Church (Old Colony Mennonite Church), 32
Russia, 22
Russlanders, use of term, 30

Salem Home (Winkler, MB), 53
Sawatzky, Leonard, 118*n*7
schizophrenia, 98, 100, 105
self-reflection, 111
sexuality, 58, 63, 65
shame, 94, 99
Simons, Menno, 21
singing events, 15
smoking, 42
Sommerfelder Church, 25, 32, 34
Southern Alberta Kanadier Association (SAKA), 9–10, 75–76
spiritual health, 42, 82, 96
spiritual illness, 44–45
stomach discomfort, 50
Strassendorf village system, 23, 25, 118*n*1
substance abuse, 42, 44–45, 101–2. *See also* alcohol and alcoholism
suffering, 45–48, 75, 83, 110
suicide, 88–89, 94

technology usage, 9, 36–37
terminology, for Low German Mennonites, 30–31
tonsillitis, 51
toothache, 49, 50
treatment: alternative health providers, 51–52, 61; assumptions about care, 50; folk remedies, 51; introduction, 48; mental health, 105–7; mixture of treatment types, 48–49, 50, 110–11; physical treatments, 49–50; religious beliefs and, 18–19, 109–11. *See also* bone-setters; lady doctor

Visser, P., 32
vomiting, 49

Waisenamt, 23, 90–91
water, anointing with, 83
Wiebe Krahn, Helena, 57

Winkler (MB), 53, 105–6
women: caregiving role, 52, 54, 61–62; clothing and appearance, 35–36, 58; family and community roles, 16, 56–57; family honour and, 63; on illness, 40; role in health care and prevention, 60
women's health: access to care, 48, 52, 60–61, 113; church's role in, 55; domestic violence, 42, 75–76; hysterectomy, 74; interview participants, 55–56; introduction and conclusions, 55–56, 76–77; lack of community support, 74; menstruation, 64–65; scholarship on, 57–60; self-care, 62–63; sexuality beliefs and understanding, 58, 63, 65. *See also* pregnancy and childbirth